Intermittent Fasting for Women Over 50

The Essential Beginner's Guide to Weight Loss, Promote Longevity, Delay Aging and Detox Your Body Through the Self-Cleansing Process of Autophagy

Table of Contents

Easy Tricks to Deceive Hunger

Proven Truths That Will Help You Maintain Your Goal

Some Examples of a Balanced Daily Meal Plan

Introduction

Congratulations on purchasing *Intermittent Fasting for Women Over 50,* and thank you for doing so.

Some of the most difficult problems after age 50 are low metabolism, joint pain, muscle mass reduction and even sleep problems. At the same time, losing fat, especially dangerous belly fat, can dramatically reduce your risk for serious health issues such as diabetes, heart attacks, and cancer. Of course, as you age, the risk of developing many diseases increases. In some cases, intermittent fasting can act as a virtual fountain of youth for women over 50 when it involves losing weight and generally reducing the likelihood of developing age-related diseases.

Intermittent fasting, often described as IF, will not force you to starve yourself. Once you do not fast, it does not give you a license to consume many unhealthy foods. Instead of eating food and snacks throughout the day, you eat within your chosen window of time.

Most people create an IF schedule, which requires them to fast for 12 to 16 hours each day. During the rest of the time, they eat normal food and snacks. Sticking to the current eating window is not as difficult as it seems because most people sleep for their eight fasting hours. Additionally, you are encouraged to enjoy the water, tea, and sometimes zero-calorie drinks.

You should develop an eating schedule that works for you for the simplest intermittent fasting results. As an example:

Twelve-hour fast: With a 12-12 fast, you will likely skip breakfast and wait until lunch. If you like to eat your morning meal, then you will eat fast and avoid evening snacks. Most older women find 12-12 fast, very easy to live.

Sixteen-hour fast: You will enjoy fast results with a 16-8 IF schedule. Most people prefer to consume two meals and a snack or two every day within an eight-hour window. For example, you would probably set your dinner window between midday and eight in the evening or between eight in the morning and 4 in the afternoon.

Five-two schedule: Restricted eating period may not work for you every day. Another option is to stay on a fast for twelve or sixteen hours for five days and then rest your schedule for two days. As an example, you could use IF during the week and normally eat on weekends.

Fasting every other day: Another variation involves very restricted calories on alternate days. For example, you will probably keep your calories below 500 at some point, then eat normally later in the day. Note that daily IF fasting never involves limiting low calories.

Some believe that IF has worked for them simply because a limited eating window naturally helps them reduce their calorie intake. For example, instead of eating three meals and two snacks, they may find that they only have two meals and snack time. They are more mindful of the types of foods they consume and tend to stay away from processed carbs, unhealthy fats, and empty calories.

Of course, you will also choose the types of healthy food that you enjoy. While some people like to reduce their overall calorie intake, others associate IF with keto, vegetarian, or other types of diets.

While some nutritionists believe that IF only works because it helps people to limit food intake naturally, others disagree. They believe that intermittent fasting with an equal number of calories and other nutrients results in better than a typical diet program. Studies have also suggested that avoiding food for several hours each day limits the number of calories you consume.

These are some metabolic changes that may help with the benefits of synergy for IF causes:

Insulin: During the fasting period, low insulin levels will help improve fat burning.

HGH: While insulin levels fall, HGH levels rise to stimulate fat burning and muscle growth.

Noradrenaline: In response to an empty stomach, the system will send this chemical to the nerve cells to let them know that they must release fat for fuel.

Is Intermittent Fasting Safe? Remember that you are purported to fast only for twelve to sixteen hours and not in a day. You still have plenty of time to enjoy a satisfying and healthy diet. Of course, some older women may have frequent meals due to metabolic disorders or prescription instructions. In this case, you should discuss your eating habits with your medical provider before making any changes.

While it is not technically fast, some doctors have reported intermittent fasting benefits by allowing such easy-to-digest food as whole fruits during the fasting window. Modifications such as these can still give your digestive and metabolic system an essential rest. For example, "Fit for Life" was a well-liked weight-loss book suggesting eating fruit after dinner and before lunch.

The of this book stated that they had patients who only changed their eating habits with this twelve-sixteen-hour "fruit" fast. They did not follow other dietary rules or count calories, and they still lost weight and were healthy. This strategy has probably worked because dieters have replaced food with whole foods. In any case, people found this dietary change to be effective and direct. Traditionalists will not call this fast; However, it is important to understand that you may have options if you absolutely cannot avoid food for several hours at a time.

Intermittent fasting, also known as intermittent energy restriction, is an umbrella term for various meal timings that is the cycle between voluntary fasting (or low-calorie intake) and non-fasting over a given period.

The three methods of intermittent fasting are alternate day fasting, periodic fasting, and daily time-restricted eating. Intermittent fasting can also be almost like a calorie restriction diet. Although being studied as an exercise within the 21st century to reduce the risk of diet-related diseases, intermittent fasting is additionally considered a fad.

There is a science competition related to intermittent fasting. The American Heart Association (AHA) states that intermittent fasting can reduce weight, reduce insulin resistance, and reduce the risk of cardiometabolic diseases, although its long-term stability is unknown. The US National Institute on Aging (NIA) specifically recommends for the elderly against intermittent fasting due to uncertainties about its effectiveness and safety. The 2019 review concluded that intermittent-fasting interventions in humans might help with obesity, insulin resistance, dyslipidemia, hypertension, and inflammation.

Alternate day fasting alternates between 24-hour "fasting days" when the person eats but accounts for 25% of normal energy needs, after that a 24-hour non-fasting "feast day" period. This is the most difficult type of intermittent fasting because there are more days of fasting per week. There are two subtypes:

Full alternate day fasting (or total intermittent energy restriction), where no calories are consumed on fasting days.

Modified alternate day-fasting (or partial, intermittent energy restriction) that allows up to 25% of daily calories consumed on fasting days rather than full fasting. This often occurs alternately with normal eating and on very low-calorie days.

Periodic fasting or full-day fasting includes any period of 24-hour continuous fasting, such as a 5: 2 diet where there are one or two fasts per week, with a fast of several days or weeks to a more extreme version. During fasting days, consumption of about 500 to 700 calories, or about 25% of the normal daily calorie intake, may be allowed instead of full fasting.

Time-restricted eating involves eating a specific number of meals every day. Skipping meals and, therefore, a 16: 8 diet (16 fasting hours cycling by eight non-fasting hours) are examples. This schedule is considered to benefit biological time.

The science related to intermittent fasting is preliminary and uncertain for the absence of studies on its future effects. Preliminary evidence indicates that intermittent fasting may also be effective for weight loss, reduce insulin resistance and fasting insulin, and should improve cardiovascular and metabolic health. However, the future stability of those effects has not been studied.

Recommendations

The recommends intermittent fasting as part of the "intentional approach to eating that focuses on the timing and frequency of food and breakfast as the basis of a healthy lifestyle and better factor management". For those who are overweight, fasting can also be integrated into a broader dietary change, such as "strategically placing snacks before meals that may be more food-related", managing appetite and controlling meal portions. Is planning meals and snacks throughout the day to assist in and promote consistency "overnight fast periods". The AHA noted that eating a few meals on an entire day (rather than a whole fast) leads to best weight loss and decreased insulin resistance when obese individuals lose a minimum of 4% weight.

The American Diabetes Association "found limited evidence about the safety and/or effect of intermittent fasting on type 1 diabetes" and did not recommend any specific dietary patterns for the management of diabetes, then preliminary results of weight loss for type 2 diabetes Until more research has been completed, it has been recommended instead that "health care providers are specialized in those key factors "Should Retry which are common between the patterns.

The New Zealand Ministry of Health believes that intermittent fasting is often recommended by doctors to some, except diabetic patients, stating that these "diets are often as effective as other energy-restricted diets, and some people may find them easier to live with "but have the potential for fasting days such as" hunger, low energy levels, mild weakness, and poor mental functioning. " Side effects occur and note that healthy food should be chosen on non-fasting days.

The NIA stated that although intermittent fasting showed weight-loss success in several studies on obese or overweight individuals, it did not recommend intermittent fasting for non-overweight individuals, especially because of uncertainty for older adults. Does.

According to the NHS choice, people considering a 5: 2 diet should consult a physician first, as fasting can sometimes be unsafe. An item within the Canadian Medical Association Journal expressed concern that publicity for the diet showed people eating high-calorie foods such as hamburgers and chips, which may have encouraged binge eating since the implication " If you fast for two days every week, you 'eat the maximum amount of waste because your gull can swallow during the remaining five days ".

Weight There is some limited evidence that intermittent fasting reduces weight like a calorie-restricted diet. Weight loss was observed in most studies on intermittent fasting in humans, ranging from 2.5% to 9.9%. Alternate day fasting does not affect lean body mass, although a review found a slight decrease. Alternate day fasting improves the cardiovascular and metabolic biomarker that is like a calorie restriction diet for overweight people who are obese or have metabolic syndrome.

Intermittent fasting has not yet been studied in children, the elderly, or underweight people, and would be harmful in these populations. Intermittent fasting is not recommended for those who are not overweight. The long-term stability of intermittent fasting was unknown as of 2018.

Other effects have been linked to poor sleep quality at nighttime eating. Intermittent fasting (prevention, treatment, drug interactions) is not recommended for the treatment of cancer in France, the UK, or the US. However, a couple of small-scale clinical studies suggest that intermittent fasting reduces chemotherapy side effects.

Fasting periodically may have a minor effect on chronic pain and mood disorders. In early research, intermittent fasting has indicated signs of reducing risk factors, certain disorders, including insulin resistance and disorders. Intermittent fasting does not affect bone health.

Adverse Effects

Early clinical studies found that short-term intermittent fasting could cause minor adverse effects, such as constant feelings of hunger, irritability, and impaired thinking. However, these effects occurred within a month of fasting exercise. Starts spreading. However, the information is sparse, as most studies have not specifically analyzed adverse effects. The 2018 systematic review found no major adverse effects. Intermittent fasting is not recommended for pregnant or lactating women during maturity, or for children and adolescents, or individuals susceptible to eating disorders.

Tolerance

Dietary Maybe a determinant of its potential effectiveness and maintenance of gaining benefits such as weight loss or biomarker improvement. The 2019 review found that intermittent varying rates varied from 2% to 38% for intermittent fasting, and from 0% to 50% for a calorie restriction diet.

Confirmatory Mechanisms

Early research indicates that fasting can induce an infection through four states: 1) During the satiated state from the tight state or absorption state when the first fuel source glucose and body fat storage is activated, approximately 4 hours lasting effect; A postabsorptive state lasting up to 18 hours when glucagon is secreted, and therefore the body uses reserves of liver glucose as a fuel source; A rapid state is transitioning rapidly to other reserves, such as fat, carboxylic acids, and alanine as fuel sources, when the liver glucose reserves are depleted, the effect occurring after 12 to 36 hours of fasting; A shift within fat deposition like free fat fatty acids from preferential lipid synthesis and fat storage metabolized into fatty acid derivative ketones to supply energy. Some call this infection a "metabolic switch". A 2019 review of the weight-change intervention, which includes alternate-day fasting, time-restricted eating, exercise, and over-eating, found that weight homeostasis cannot fix for "energetic errors" loss or gain of calories in short-term.

Intermittent Feeding

Other feeding schemes, such as hypocaloric feeding and intermittent feeding, also known as bolus feeding, were studied. A 2019 meta-analysis found that intermittent feeding may be more beneficial for premature infants. However, better-designed studies are needed to plan clinical practices. In adults, reviews have not received intermittent feeding to expand glucose variability or gastrointestinal intolerance. A meta-analysis found that intermittent feeding had no effect on gastric residual volumes and aspiration, pneumonia, mortality, or morbidity in people with stroke, but increased the risk of diarrhea.

History

Fasting is an ancient tradition practiced by many cultures and religions for centuries.

Medical intermittent fasting for the treatment of obesity has been investigated since at least 1915, with renewed interest in the medical profession within the 1960s after Bloom and his colleagues published an "enthusiastic report". Intermittent fasting, or "periods of short-term starvation," were beginning in these early studies from 1 to 14 days. This enthusiasm entered Late Magazine, which prompted researchers and clinicians to exercise caution about the use of intermittent fasting with medical monitoring.

The 5:2 diet, a modern type of intermittent fasting, began in the UK in 2012.

Religious Fasting

Intermittent fasting is practiced in religious practices throughout the planet. These include Vat (Hinduism), Ramadan (Islam), Yom Kippur and other fasts (Judaism), Orthodox Christian fasting, Sundays (the Church of Jesus of the saints), and Buddhist fasting. Religious fasting practices may only require restraint from certain foods or (Yom Kippur), which last for a short period of your time and produce negligible effects.

In Buddhism, fasting Theravada is performed as a part of the monastic training of Buddhist monks, who fast daily from noon to midday sunrise. This daily fasting pattern can also be made by pruning after eight sermons.

During Ramadan, Islamic practices are almost like intermittent fasting by not eating or drinking from dawn to sunset, while consuming food before dawn and after dusk within the evening. A meta-analysis on the health of Muslims during Ramadan shows significant weight loss during the fasting period of up to 1.51 kg (3.3 lb.). Still, this weight was regained within about a fortnight after that. The analysis concluded that

"Ramadan offers a chance to reduce, but structured and consistent lifestyle modifications are necessary to realize lasting weight loss." One review found similarities between Ramadan and time-restricted food, with the greatest disparity being the lack of drinking water with Islamic fasting. The negative effects of fasting Ramadan increase the risk of hypoglycemia in diabetic patients, as well as insufficient levels of certain nutrients.

Chapter 1: Weight Gain and Eating Problems in Women

Eating disorders, especially anorexia and bulimia nervosa, have been classically described in young women in Western populations. Recent research suggests that they are also seen in developing countries, including India. The classification of eating disorders has recently been expanded to include conditions such as binge eating disorder. There is a multifunctional etiology in eating disorders. Genetic factors play a serious role. Recent advances in neurobiology have improved our understanding of those conditions. They should possibly help us develop simpler treatments in the future. Premorbid personality plays an important role, with differences for individual disorders. The role of cultural factors is debated within the etiology of those situations. Culture may have a path plastic effect that results in non-presentation of non-fat-like non-fatty types of anorexia, which are commonly reported in developing countries. With the rapid cultural change, these types of classical types are being described throughout the planet. Diagnostic criteria have been revised for these numerous presentations. Treatments for eating disorders are often quite challenging, given the established treatments and poor motivation/lack of insight into these conditions. Nutrition remains the mainstay of rehabilitation and psychotherapeutic treatment, while pharmacotherapy may also be helpful in specific situations.

At the end of the 17th century, for the first time, cases of caries without medical reason occurred. The term anorexia was introduced by William Google in 1874 to explain four cases of teenage girls deliberately losing weight. Weight phobia, which is taken to be central to the concept of eating disorders, was described as characteristic of eating disorders only within the 1930s. Therefore, some (but not all) suggest that weight loss may also be an artwork created by cultural changes in the 1930s and should not be the main feature of the disorder.

Russell first described bulimia nervosa in 1979 as an "ominous version of anorexia". Later descriptions have shown bulimia nervosa to be an independent disorder, with traditional weight-eating behavior. Some have hypothesized that bulimia nervosa was nothing before recent times, and changes in cultural and economic conditions, such as increased prosperity and surplus of food, have led to the onset of the disorder. Others have presented historical cases with possible bulimia nervosa to suggest that the disorder may be present but not identified at earlier times. However, KL and Klomp, who systematically reviewed historical cases, suggest that these were close to binge disorder (BED); Bulimia nervosa is probably a culture-bound syndrome of recent origin.

In developing countries, anorexia was rarely reported until the 1970s and 1980s. But later studies have confirmed the presence of eating disorders; A number of these studies suggest that the prevalence of eating disorders may be almost even within Western countries. However, in non-Western countries, patients often present without major weight concerns.

Most Common Eating Disorders

Based on similarities in psychotherapy and higher, many have tried to classify eating disorders as subtypes of mood, obsessive-compulsive or mental disorders, etc. However, eating disorders are "true to the breed", and a mood. Or other disorders. Within the International Classification of Disease Classification 10 (ICD 10), eating disorders are considered independently and classified under the broad category of "behavioral disturbances related to physical disturbances and physiological factors".

Anorexia nervosa and bulimia nervosa are the main eating disorders included within the Diagnostic and Statistical Manual of Mental Disorders, 4th ed., Text Revision (DSM-IV-TR). Additionally, ICD 10 includes "vomiting related to other psychiatric disturbances", "atypical anorexia," "atypical bulimia nervosa", and "related to other psychiatric disturbances under eating disorders". In DSM-IV-TR, anorexia is subtyped in binge-eating/purging type and restricted type. Bulimia nervosa is reduced to purging and no purging types. In the DSM-IV-TR, BED is included in the appendix as a qualifying condition for further study.

Studies have shown that the bulk of patients with the disorder fit into the unnecessary category of eating disorder unless otherwise specified (EDNOS). The validity of this category as a clinical entity has been questioned; Because it also includes subtype types of anorexia, bulimia nervosa as other disorders that do not fit into these categories. ICD 10 partially covers the subtype of disorders, including atypical anorexia and atypical bulimia nervosa. Recent research set out to find clinically useful and nosologically valid entities within the EDNOS group; For example, BYD, night eating syndrome, purging syndrome, etc. Purging disorder is seen in normal-weight individuals who induce themselves by vomiting or laxatives in the absence of binge eating. Night Eating Syndrome is characterized by large amounts of food, with already dark-related sleep and morning anorexia.

The inclusion of BED and obesity is under active consideration of the DSM-V Working Group. However, current evidence suggests that obesity may be a condition of heterogeneous etiology. There is evidence that obesity is usually caused by mental illness.

Korean features have been debated in the improved amenorrhea as a criterion for anorexia. It is considered useful because it is clear and objective. Also, the presence of amenorrhea may reflect important biological abnormalities that provide information about the etiology of the disease and/or may inform the occurrence of biological treatments. But studies have shown that many patients meet all diagnostic criteria for anorexia in addition to amenorrhea. Most of the differences between patients with and without amenorrhea reflect the nutritional status of the patient, rather than any major pathology. So, various advocate removal of amenorrhea as an important criterion for the diagnosis of anorexia.

Patients suffering from Fat phobia uncontrolled reports from non-Western countries with findings showed symptoms ranging from those who present variously to the refusal of food, aside from weight concerns. Ann is credited with portraying this phenomenological form of anorexia. Lee et al. Investigated the pathology of 70 Chinese patients with anorexia in Hong Kong. But one-half of the patients were found to report fat fear at some point during their illness. Instead, weight loss mainly consisted of flatulence, loss of appetite, fear of food, or eating less. The concluded that "fatphobia, cross-culturally speaking, is not a prison for all cases of morbid self-starvation" and proposed that "the identification of anorexia envisaged without affecting the specifically interpretive construct of fat" Should be done. ". "A series of 5 cases without anxiety has also been reported in India. Such patients with low weight concerns are seen in about 15–20% of cases of eating disorders within Western countries. It has also been seen That South Asians living in Western countries are less frequently present with Fat Phobia than the White English population. However, the Eating Disorders "Drive for Thinness" sub-center Studies conducted to isolate patients without weight concerns and anxiety suggest that patients with low scores on the "drive for thinness" have lower morbidity than patients with higher scores and is common psychopathology. Also, a fat phobia may be supported during treatment. Therefore, while many theorists have been diagnosed with anorexia as "weight f Has advocated the removal of the criterion". Others suggested that weight phobia is the sign qualification of anorexia nervosa is nonsignificant and will remain intact within future diagnostic systems. Supporting a scientific review, Baker et al. Explain that non-fat phobic anorexia as a subtype of anorexia does not meet the criteria for robins and diagnostic validity. However, thanks to its frequent presentation in various countries, they suggest its inclusion as a standardized presentation of EDNOS to strengthen its clinical description.

Clinical features the clinical features of Eating disorders are diverse and usually involve multiple body systems. However, the major symptoms are related to eating, weight, and size.

Anorexia Nervosa

Several criteria are proposed for the diagnosis of anorexia. Most standards share the latter's essential features:

Weight loss/weight reduction and behavior deficiencies that are designed to supply such weight loss.

A psychopath characterized by a relentless drive for thinness and/or fear of obese morbidity. Essential psychopathology seems to be primarily associated with the prevalence of thinness to more prevalent beliefs. The drive for thinness as a psychopathological motif has been emphasized more by Americans, starting with Hilde Bruch, while the fear of obesity, avoiding the normal weight phobic, British emphasis is more emphasized by

The medical consequences starvation: Examples of Endocrine dysfunction. Appearing as amenorrhea in women and decreased sexual strength in men, hypothermia, bradycardia, orthostasis, and decrease in body fat stores, etc.

Anorexia nervosa usually, but not always, is related to disturbances of body image, the notion that a person is troubled is huge despite apparent medical starvation. Distortion of body image is disturbed when present but is not necessary for pathognomonic, invisibility, or diagnosis.

ICD 10 applies the following criteria for the diagnosis of anorexia nervosa:

Weight loss or, in children, loss of weight gain, resulting in at least 15% less traditional or expected weight for age or height.

The loss is self-induced by avoiding "fast foods".

There is a self-perception of being too fat, with a terrible fear of obesity, resulting in a voluntary low weight threshold. Pervasive endocrine disorder in the hypothalamic-pituitary-gonadal axis manifests as amenorrhea in women and a lack of sexual interest and potency in men (an obvious exception is vaginal bleeding in anorexic women who replace hormonal replacements While on therapy, mostly taken in the form of a contraceptive pill) the

The disorder does not. Standards for bulimia nervosa do not meet A and B.

Bulimia Nervosa

There are recurrent episodes of overfeeding, during which a short intake of large amounts of food is taken because of a strong desire for food and a great craving to eat.

the patient attempts to counteract the "fattening" effects of food, with one or more of these modes:

-Self-induced vomiting

-Self-induced purification

-Alternative periods of starvation

-Use of medication like appetite suppressants, thyroid preparations, or diuretics; When diabetic patients have bulimia, they would prefer to neglect their insulin treatment.

-There is a self-perception of being very fat, which has a terrible fear of obesity (usually resulting in weight loss).

Patients with bulimia nervosa have a strong and attractive urge to fill the stomach and a lack of control over binge-eating episodes. There are controversies regarding the standards for what constitutes a binge. Some specialize in food counts, some on the subjective state of Man et al. At a rapid rate of eating. The DSM-IV gives your "eating," criterion during a discrete period (for example, within a 2-h period), a similar period and in similar circumstances will eat a larger amount than most people "and one Lack of in-kind control. The clinical features of bulimia nervosa are almost like those of binge eating/purification of anorexia. These disorders often result in massive weight loss in patients with anorexia. It is different from the appearance.

Binge Disorder

BED is characterized by recurrent episodes of vomiting or laxative abuse, such as binge eating in the absence of the normal compensatory behavior. Related features include uncomfortably full of food when not physically hungry Eating, eating alone, and feeling of depression or guilt.

Although it is not limited to obese individuals, it is most common during this group and those who I ask for treatment of overweight rather than more food. The prevalence of Bed is reported to be 2 to 5% in community samples and 30% in individuals seeking weight control treatment. It is bulimia. It has a more equal sex ratio than Nervosa. BED disorder is related to increased psychotherapy, including depression and personality disorders.

Comorbidity Moving

Clinical challenges of disorders to be identified by a handful of eating disorders are partially Ptah an, because, in most cases, Comorbid psychiatric disorders. Common co-occurring conditions include:

Mood/Affective Disorder

It is commonly seen in patients with both anorexia and bulimia nervosa. Recent studies have shown a high degree of sympathy between bipolar affective disorders and eating disorders, particularly between bulimia nervosa and bipolar II disorders. This symbiosis becomes more pronounced when disorders are included.

Anxiety

disorders disorder is generally more prevalent in people with hysteria prevalence and obsessive-compulsive disorder, especially those with anorexia and bulimia nervosa. Anxiety disorders often have their onset in childhood before the onset of a disorder, supporting the possibility that they are a vulnerability factor for the development of anorexia or bulimia nervosa.

Substance abuse disorders are associated with an increased risk of multiple substance use disorders, the risk being greater for bulimia nervosa, and subtype epilogue of binge eating/anorexia.

Personality Traits and Disorders

It has been suggested that anorexia may also be associated with observational and perfectionistic types of physical disturbances, bulimia nervosa with impulsive and unstable personality disorders, and avoidance of personality disorders and BED with anxious types. Cluster B and personality disorder are reported to predict a poor course and/or outcome, and hysteric personality traits and self-directedness are reported to predict a more favorable course and/or outcome. Within the setting of a disorder, weak personality traits can also be manifested as primary personality disorders, but secondary personality disturbances.

Other Psychopathological Disorders

There is elevated comorbidity of anorexia with body debility disorder, estimated at 25–39% - during which patients do not have observations about specific body parts specifically associated with weight or size.

Pathology

The results from medical complications in eating disorders (a) amount and rate of starvation, (b) means to produce weight loss (with or without exercise alone, self-induced vomiting, laxatives, diet pills diuretics), And (c) binge eating.

In patients with anorexia, each major organ system is often involved, and therefore the risk of mortality is substantial. Particular areas of concern are dermatologic changes (some of which require acute intervention; egg, purpura), endocrine abnormalities (including diabetic mismanagement), gastrointestinal problems (including gastrointestinal hazards), cardiovascular/pulmonary problems (arrhythmia and Including pneumomediastinum)), severe electrolyte abnormalities, and bone excretion.

Eating disorders are associated with one of the best rates of mortality among psychiatric disorders, up to 19% within 20 years of hospitalization, starting at 20. Disorder patients either die from the medical consequences of starvation (loss and arrhythmias of the heart muscle, sometimes associated with hypokalemia) or suicide. During a meta-analysis conducted in 1995 out of 42 published studies, crude mortality was 5.9%, which changed to 0.56% / year or 5.6% per decade. Explaining the explanation of death in the study, 54% of patients died as a result of abstinence complications, 27% committed suicide, and so the remaining 19% died of unknown or other causes. During a meta-analysis of standardized mortality (SMR) in 2001, anorexia had a normal total SMR of 9.6 in follow-up studies of 6 to 12 years and studies with 3.7 in 20–40 years of follow-up. Anorexia comorbid correlates with alcohol dependence up to 50 times higher, and anorexia comorbid with insulin-dependent DM alone with a 10-fold higher mortality rate in those diseases.

Epidemiology Western countries incident have used psychiatric case registers or medical records of hospitals in besieged areas in most detailed studies of eating disorders. Therefore, they underestimate the events within the community. The reported incidence of anorexia and bulimia nervosa is 8 / 100,000 person/year and 13 / 100,000 person/year, respectively. Studies including a meta-analysis in Western cultures suggest that the incidence of anorexia increased until 1970 when it reached a plateau.

Prevalence

Based on National Comet Survey replication, lifetime prevalence estimates of anorexia, bulimia nervosa, and BYD are estimated at 0.9%, 1.5%, and 3.5%, respectively, in women and 0.3%, 0.5%, and 2.0% in men. Other researchers suggest that only 15% of people have no prejudice with dieting, weight, or size; Therefore, sub-disorders of eating behavior may also be more prevalent. Psychiatry is one of the most important gender-deviation disorders, but deviations are already considered. Previous estimates of the ratio of men to women for eating disorders were typically 1 to 10 in 20–1. Recent community-based epidemiological studies, however, found ratios of about 3 to 1 for both anorexia and bulimia nervosa.

Non-Western Countries

earlier suggested in the study that anorexia was rare in non-Western countries, including India. A prevalence rate of 0.02–0.03% has been

31

observed in epidemiological studies in Korea. Nakamura et al. A prevalence of 0.003% was found in the general population, and anorexia nervosa in 0.005% of the female population; And 1.02 / 100,000 women had bulimia nervosa during an operational area in Japan. Kuroki et al.

Prevalence was found to be three in 1985 and two for eating disorders. 9–3.7 / 100,000 and in Japan in 1992 was three .6–4.5 / 100,000 for anorexia and 1.3–2.5 / 100,000 for bulimia nervosa. Azuma and Hemi found a rural/urban difference with a prevalence of 0.2% in urban areas and 0.05% in rural areas. Chen et al. Hong Kong were found to have a prevalence of 0.03%. No bat and Duckham reported a prevalence of 0.9% for anorexia and three .2% for bulimia nervosa in high school students in Iran. Prevalence of 0.9% in Egypt and 0.002% for bulimia nervosa in Pakistan was found among high school students. Also, they noted the increasing prevalence of eating disorders related to body dissatisfaction in non-Western countries, presumed to have an effect of Westernization. Studies in Western countries show that eating disorders are more frequent among ethnic minorities.

In their review of studies in non-Western countries, Keel and Klomp commented, "Anorexia represents a similar proportion of the overall and psychiatric population in many Western and non-Western countries, except for the criterion of weight concerns." There was a relatively small difference in the prevalence of bulimia nervosa and anorexia in non-Western countries compared to Western countries. They hypothesize that bulimia is culturally more dependent than anorexia.

Risk Factors

Currently, eating disorders are regarded as complex disorders with etiology, which include biological, psychological, and environmental factors, such as most other psychiatric syndromes.

Biological facts Since the late 19th century, when eating disorders were thought to arise from postpartum pituitary necrosis, biological principles for eating disorders were hip. Although this theory was soon disproved, a proliferation of later theories has advanced that specialize in curative biological undergrowth - for example, there exists some preconceived hypothalamic abnormality, evident by amenorrhea. However, recent evidence suggests that endocrine abnormalities result from starvation. The current biological hypothesis suggests that eating disorders represent a pathology and is controlled by traditional neuroscience redundancy that regulates eating behavior in response to a sustained drive for thinness and a fear conditioning about normal weight.

Recent evidence has shown a strong genetic contribution to the etiology of eating disorders. Twin studies exhibit 3 times more symmetry in monozygotic twins than in monogamous twins. Genetic factors such as anorexia and bulimia nervosa can contribute significantly to 50%. Large studies have shown a consistent (but not exclusive) link between the 5-HT (2A) receptor gene and, therefore, the BDNF gene and polymorphic variants limiting the subtype to anorexia. Anderson and

Yage suggest that genetic factors likely contribute by increasing the presence and potency of risk factors, such as persistence, perfectionist, sensitive, fearful, or impulsive personality traits, or through biological weaknesses that are more easily ingested. It causes serotonergic mechanisms to be disrupted.

Contemporary theories point to the therapeutic serotonin mechanism, supporting comments that individuals with anorexia have abnormal spinal serotonin levels when they are ill, which will not partially reverse completely when weight gain occurs. Using a 5-HT specific ligand, brain imaging studies suggest that disturbances of 5-HT function occur when people are ill and persist after recovery from anorexia and bulimia nervosa. It has been postulated that characteristic disturbances of 5-HT neuronal modulation occur before the onset of anorexia and affect the symptoms of hysteria, obsessiveness, and inhibition. Other neuromodulators such as disturbed corticotropin-releasing hormones, opioids, cholecystokinin, neuropeptide Y, peptide YY, leptin, Grain, etc. have also been implicated in the etiology of eating disorders.

Neuroimaging studies suggest that eating disorders cause a decrease in think alba and gray matter volume but are reminiscent of recovery. Studies have implicated the cingulate, frontal, temporal, and parietal regions in anorexia. Functional studies suggest that challenges such as food and body image distortions can activate many of these areas. These disturbances persist after recovering from anorexia, raising the possibility that these symptoms may also be neighborhoods of vulnerability to developing disorders.

Archaeological Factors In the second half of the 20th century, psychiatric formulations of eating disorders were predicted. Early yoga was focused on the fear of verbal impregnation. However, they were replaced by yoga emphasizing additive and existential fears. Restricting one type of anorexia, as well as providing shocks that evoke a negative reaction to emerging sexuality and other biological and social challenges of adolescence.

Childhood presence of symptoms such as perfectionism, rigor, and rule-bounding increase the risk of developing anorexia by an element of about seven each. Trauma during childhood or adolescence contributes to the possibility of later psychiatric disorders, usually, not exclusively disorders.

Investigators are beginning to identify endophenotypes, such as poor set-shifting and weak central coherence, with the help of family studies. These can help uncover the psychology of eating disorders.

Environmental Manufacturers

Keel and Klomp comment that anorexia has a pathogenic effect about anxiety in weight, whereas bulimia nervosa seems to be a culture-bound syndrome. Weight loss is found in many cases from non-Western countries.

To see whether eating disorders are etiologically associated with the internalization of social pressure, which arises from the standards of female greatness about fashionable industrial society or Western culture, of the current discourse around the etiology of eating disorders. It occupies a prominent position within. Environmental factors such as enrollment in ballet schools, teasing by family and friends, and comments and authority from authority figures (doctors, nurses, teachers, coaches) about changing statistics play a function within the pathogenesis of eating disorders.

Lee suggests that appreciation of thinness is not inherent to non-Western cultures. Kayenta et al. Comparison of body dissatisfaction and eating attitudes among students of Indian (living in Muscat, Oman), Omani, Filipino, Japanese, and Euro-American backgrounds. Subjects in India, Oman, and therefore the Philippines exhibited almost the same or worse eating than subjects in Western countries and Japan. Still, their desire for thinness was not as strong. Studies have shown that although non-Western cultures have degraded eating behavior, it is likely to be driven by reasons different from body dissatisfaction. However, globalization and exposure to Western media can increase the speed of eating disorders in non-Western countries. Recent studies in Fiji suggest that popular television programs revealed early obesity, reducing slimness and stigma, which introduced widespread dietary behavior and led to the emergence of the latest cases of eating disorders in the population that Previously unaffiliated with these issues.

Westernization is not the only cultural factor playing an etiological role in eating disorders. In some studies, ethnic minorities in Westernized countries have increased disordered eating behaviors (as measured by eating attitudes test scores); And the relationship between disorganized eating behavior and a "traditional" South Asian cultural orientation. It was envisaged that integration into Western society promoted difficulties in eating behavior. However, even this evidence indicates the importance of cultural factors within the pathogenesis of eating disorders, while making it clear that quite a cultural factor may play a function.

The hazards of eating management the main treatment goals for all eating disorders are as follows:

Achieving and maintaining a traditional, healthy, individual, stable body weight.

Stopping all abnormal eating behaviors, such as restricting food, binge eating, or purging, and associated unusual behaviors, especially compulsive exercise.

Dismissing the original overvalued beliefs and unhealthy cognitive "schema" of automatic cognitive distortions, replacing them with healthy, self-balanced thoughts (not primarily bending overweight or size) and, therefore, emotional and behavioral self-regulation ability.

Treating comorbid conditions, psychiatry, and medicine, and to plan for prevention to continue for about five years after rapid improvement.

Management of eating disorders begins with the formation of a therapeutic alliance, followed by comprehensive psychotherapy and medical evaluation (including body index). The requirement for laboratory analysis should be determined on a private basis. Bone density examinations should be obtained for patients who are hemorrhagic for six months or longer.

The severity of the disease in the treatment plan should match the intensity of treatment. The choice of whether the patient should be hospitalized on a psychiatric versus a general medical or juvenile/pediatric unit should be supported by the patient's general medical and psychiatric status, the talent of the local psychiatric and general medical staff and Skills, and therefore the availability of appropriate programs to concern the patient's general medical and mental problems.

Treatment methods include medical, nutritional, educational, psychotherapy, behavioral, and pharmacological components.

Nutrition Rehabilitation

The nutritional rehabilitation for goals of seriously underweight patients are to achieve normal patterns of eating normal patterns, reviving weight, hunger and satiety, and proper biological and psychological sequelae of malnutrition. The initial short-term goal is to completely, safely resuscitate patients and immediately reach healthy limits, as determined by age, height, and gender or weight at which menstrual withdrawal for adolescents 50 % have a chance. Girls. Caloric intake should be done cautiously to avoid the syndrome. The calorie intake level should usually start at 30–40 kcal/kg/day (about 1000–1600 kcal/day). During the load regain phase, the intake may need to be progressively elevated to 70–100 kcal/kg/day for some patients.

Pharmacotherapy

Antidepressants, antipsychotics, anticonvulsants, prokinetic agents, opium, appetite suppressants, tetrahydrocannabinol, cyproheptadine, zinc, and ondansetron are tested for the treatment of eating disorders. Available evidence suggests that fluoxetine may also be beneficial in preventing anorexia after weight loss. Cyproheptadine has been shown to possess some minor benefits within the weight restoration phase of anorexia treatment. Antidepressants, particularly selective serotonin reuptake inhibitors, at an improved dose (egg, 60 mg fluoxetine) may also be useful within the treatment of bulimia nervosa and BED.

Psychotherapy

Psychotherapies are key elements of treatment aimed at modifying and changing core pathological beliefs and contributing to psychopathological issues. The available evidence is strongly in favor of therapies supporting cognitive-behavioral therapies (CBT). Anorexia patients also react with CBT without weight concerns. Additional alternative psychotherapeutic interventions supported interpersonal therapies, family therapies, or psychologically informed psychotherapies - particularly those using self-psychology and "focal analytical" approaches - may also be beneficial.

Some Studies on Food

Food enthusiasts and Awadhi in India were probably primary to report a case of disorder in India. They describe a 42-year-old woman's case of self-induced starvation of three weeks duration with the assumption that fasting will improve her memory. He did not possess any weight concerns or body image disturbances. The case report did not mention the extent of weight loss and history regarding amenorrhea. Nicki et al. Reported a pair of identical twins, aged 15, who presented with food rejection, loss of weight, and amenorrhea.

There was also a lack of body image disturbances in these cases. Chadha et al. Reported a case of anorexia, which met DSM-III criteria, during a 13-year-old woman with comrade systemic lay. The disease began after parents and siblings taunted the patient about their steroid-induced weight gain. Khandelwal et al. reported a case series of 5 patients with multiple features of anorexia but no disturbances in body image. Then there are recent reports of binge/purification of anorexia and bulimia nervosa.

Epidemiology

Although some have commented that anorexia is not as rare in India as before, no general population study has been conducted in India. Some studies have eliminated special populations, but most of them have relied on self-report inventions (for case identification) or chart review. Bhangra and Raja have questioned the applicability of self-report tools for eating approaches in non-Western cultures when no attempt is made to determine the defendants' understanding of the usually subtle and Western orientation of many questions.

Srinivasan et al Studied 210 medical students with standardized instruments. They found that no scholar could be diagnosed as having anorexia or bulimia nervosa. However, about 15% of the scholars were suffering from a subclinical disorder called "Eating Distress Syndrome."

Bhangra et al. A study was conducted on 504 students in an all-girls private college in an industrial city in North India using the Hindi translation of the Bulimic Investigatory Test, Edinburgh. They found that two patients above the cutoff for bulimia nervosa gave a prevalence of about 0.4%.

Mail carriers et al. Conducted a retrospective chart review of youth and adolescents (

Eating disorders destroying mental illnesses that affect an estimated 20 million American women and 10 million American men over their lifetime. About 85 percent to 95 percent of people who eat Disorders suffer from anorexia. And bulimia nervosa are women.

However, eating disorders revolve around eating and weight gain., They are often more about control, emotions, and self-expression about food. Women with eating disturbances often use food and diet as a way of coping with life. Stress. For some people, Food becomes a source of rest and nutrition, or how to regulate or release stress. For others, losing weight may begin with how friends and family feel about approval. Eating disorder anorexia is not a sign of personal. Weakness or problems are that the proper treatment without.

Eating disorders are completely socioeconomic and ethnic groups. 12 to 25 years old Girls in. Because of the shame associated with this complex disease, many women do not seek treatment nor seek help for years. Eating disorders also occur in young children, older women, and men, but much less frequently.

Four dietary disorders are diagnosed: anorexia, bulimia nervosa, binge disorder and disorder not otherwise specified (EDN).

Anorexia can be a disorder during which dieting and thinning result in excess weight loss. If you are suffering from the disease, you will not accept that losing weight or restricted eating can be a problem. When you are attenuated, you will still "feel fat". Women with anorexia intentionally starve themselves or exercise excessively during a relentless effort to slim down, reducing their normal weight by about 15 percent. Almost all women affected by anorexia never return to their pre-anorexic health, and about 20 percent remain chronically ill. The death rate for anorexia is better than any psychiatric. Deaths are equally divided between medical complications associated with suicide and starvation.

Women with bulimia regularly and sometimes secretly binge on large amounts of food - often between 2,000 and 5,000 calories at a time and on rare occasions, even twenty, 000 at a time Calories - then experience intense feelings of guilt or shame and scrutiny. Out to compensate by getting surplus calories. Some people are motivated by vomiting, laxatives, and diuretics or taking enemas. Others fast or exercise to extremes. If you are suffering from the disease, you are feeling out of control and recognize that your behavior is not normal, but often deny to others that you have a drag. Women who have bulimia are often of normal weight or overweight and should experience weight fluctuations.

Women with binge disorder (BED) also bid on large amounts of food for brief periods. Still, unlike women with bulimia, they are not using weight control behaviors, such as reducing a binge session or Fasting or purification in an attempt to catch up. When the binge is over, a private with BYD will often feel extreme disgust, guilty and depression about overeating.

The fourth type of disorder, the disorder not otherwise specified, refers to symptoms that do not fit the opposite three eating disorders. Individuals with EDNOS may have elements of BED or maybe on the verge of diagnosis of anorexia or bulimia, but do not meet the full diagnostic criteria. EDNOS is just a term for anyone with significant eating problems that do not meet the standards for an opposite diagnosis. Most of those who seek treatment for eating disorders fall into this category.

Although it is synonymous with eating disorders, anorexia is comparatively rare, affecting between 0.5 percent and 1 percent of girls over their lifetime, consistent with the National Alliance on Mental Disease. Another 2 percent to three percent develop bulimia and three .5 percent develop binge disorder.

Nevertheless, the figures do not tell the full story. More women, who do not necessarily meet all the standards for the disorder, are preoccupied with their bodies and are caught in a destructive pattern of dieting and overwriting, which will severely affect their health and well-being.

There is not a single explanation for eating disorders. Biological, social and psychological factors all perform a function. Evidence suggesting a genetic trend suggests that anorexia may also be more common among sisters and identical twins. Therefore, a woman with a mother or sister who has anorexia is 12 times more likely than the overall public to develop that disorder and four times more likely to develop bulimia. Furthermore, in identical twins, whose genetic makeup is equal to one hundred pcs, there is a 59 percent probability that if a twin child has anorexia, the opposite twin will also develop a disorder. For fraternal twins who share only 50 percent of their twin siblings' genes, there is an 11 percent probability that the opposite twin will have the disorder.

Other research points to hormonal disturbances and imbalances of neurotransmitters, chemicals within the brain that regulate mood and appetite, among other things.

In some women, a series or series of events trigger the disorder and allow it to take root and flourish. Triggers are often as subtle as a derogatory comment or as painful as rape or incest. Infection times, such as puberty, divorce, marriage, or early college, can also provoke disorderly eating behaviors. Parents who are over or concerned about the weight of a daughter before eating and coaches, and coaches who reliably apply weigh-ins or a particular body image to their athletes, especially weight-conscious sports such as In ballet, cheering, diving, wrestling, and gymnastics. May also inadvertently encourage a disorder. Additionally, the pressure to live during a culture where self-worth is equated with unattainable standards of thinness and surprise can also eliminate body image and / or eating issues.

Furthermore, the discrepancy between our society's concept of "ideal" body shape for women and, therefore, the size of the typical American woman has never been greater - leading many women to unrealistic goals where weight gain occurs.

Diagnosis

Because the consequences of eating disorders are often severe, early diagnosis is important for permanent recovery. Eating disorders can typically inhibit physical and emotional development in adolescents and cause premature osteoporosis. In this condition, bones become weak and more likely to fracture. Additionally, there is a risk of hormonal imbalance as a result of osteoporosis, amenorrhea and disordered eating behavior, which may also contribute to a better risk of infertility and miscarriage.

Anorexia Nervosa, a severe, potentially life-threatening disease characterized by self-starvation and excessive weight loss, is the best mortality rate of any mental disease. It usually begins in early to mid-adolescence and is one of the most common psychiatric conditions in young people seeking treatment. Among the physical effects of anorexia are:

Anemia, often caused by iron deficiency, which reduces the ability of the blood to hold oxygen and causes fatigue, difficulty breathing, dizziness, headache, insomnia, pale skin., decrease in appetite and irregular

To increase the height of cholesterol heart, which affects the function of the eating disorders liver is because, steroids Generating reduce secretion Which will enable more cholesterol to remain within the body rather than the cholesterol Korhonen and reduced and low blood heat and cold hands and legs constipation atria vital signs slow metabolism and reverse slow Pulse, which can be mistaken as a fitness symbol, due to irregular heartbeat, which can cause slowing down and cognitive and mood swings.

By the time the secondary turns to starvation, there is an intense fear of becoming fat in women with anorexia and, therefore, is inclined to food, body shape, and size. For example, for women with anorexia, it is common to gather recipes and prepare gourmet meals for family and friends. Still, it should not consume any food by themselves. Instead, they allow their bodies to reduce their appetite and "disappear" as a measure of their control. Women are struggling with anorexia diet because they need to increase their self-esteem and feelings of love not to lose a pound or two. Depression and insomnia are often accompanied by eating disorders.

Women struggling with anorexia can confine their emotions to themselves, rarely disregard authority, and are often described as perfectionists. These individuals are often good students and excellent athletes. Anorexia is common among dancers and competitive athletes in sports such as gymnastics and ice skating, where success is measured not only on athletic performance but also on having an "ideal" body.

May include symptoms of anorexia are:

- Distorted body image and weight gain Kiladar

- Menstrual irregularities

- Excessive body / facial hair

- Compulsive exercise

- Bulimia nervosa

Fear excessive using bulimia emotionally calming or soothing food and food Nervosa. How binge gets to reduce stress, anxiety, or depression. Self-induced vomiting, purgative calorie through laxative or diuretic misuse or over-exercise, relieves the guilt of overeating, and even how emotional stress or tension is until the emotional stress cycle becomes a habit Should leave. Women who have bulimia are generally more impulsive, more socially outgoing and exhibit less self-control than those who suffer from anorexia. They are more likely to abuse alcohol and other substances.

Only 6 percent of these warring bulimia receive psychiatric state care. Eating disorders are incredibly latent illnesses, and so symptoms are often hidden or appear subtle, even to friends and loved ones. For example, women battling bulimia are not necessarily thin; They will be at an average weight and even a touch bit overweight.

Nevertheless, they will remain nutritionally hungry as they are not getting vitamins, minerals, and other nutrients.

Symptoms of bulimia include:

- Problems with food, weight, and appearance

- Binge eating, usually secretly

- Vomiting and excessive use of colds or diuretics

- Menstrual irregularities

- Mandatory exercise is among

The physical effects of bulimia:

- Dehydration

- Chronic diarrhea

- Excessive weakness

- Intestines and liver congestion renal content

Electrolyte imbalance and low potassium Diffusers, which cause irregular heartbeat, and in some cases, due to repeated stomach acid exposure to the stomach, contact with broken blood vessels within the eyes and swollen glands on the face. wrinkles have who is self-motivated and may be indicated vomiting Keleti cause self-inflicted Unties toes cuts and Colors,

The fifth edition of the Diagnostic and Statistical Manual of Mental Disorders (DSM), released in 2013, recognized BYD as a political disorder.

Like bulimia, people with BED engage in binge eating or rapid consumption of large amounts of food. Still, they also compensate for behaviors such as fasting or purging to "undo" the consequences of binge eating and control their weight. Are not using. People with BED eat large amounts of food, even when they are not hungry. They struggle to differentiate between physical and emotional hunger, feel uncomfortable after eating, and sometimes feel distressed about their binge sessions.

Like the other two official eating disorders, BYD can occur with other psychiatric disorders, such as depression, drug abuse, or anxiety disorders. Over time, women with BED realize thanks to being overweight, so the disorder is usually (but not always) related to obesity.

If BYD is left untreated, it can lead to obesity, which can lead to its medical the results are such as:

- High Vital Signs

- High Cholesterol

- Gallbladder Disease

- Diabetes

- Heart Disease

- Some Types of Cancer

- Tests for Eating Disorder Eating disorder

Complicated There are mental illnesses, and there is no medical test that will diagnose a disorder. However, when you are seeking treatment for disorders, your health care professional can work to remove several of your blood if you are affected by any medical outcome associated with a disorder. Here are some things that will be tested:

electrolyte balance. It checks primarily for dehydration but can also be a sign of malnutrition due to self-induced vomiting or laxative or diuretic abuse. Electrolytes are a selected combination of minerals that your body must maintain to function properly, such as sodium and potassium. Common symptoms of imbalance are leg cramps, heart palpitations, high or low vital symptoms and swelling within the legs and feet. Electrolyte imbalance can lead to kidney failure, attack, and even death.

B12 and Vitamin BC intake assessment. B12 and vitamin BC deficiency may be caused by, or caused by, the metabolism of proteins, carbohydrates, and fats, and by the body's ability to absorb nutrients. Low levels of B12 or vitamin BC can contribute to depression and anxiety.

Blood sugar level: Low levels of blood sugar are often the result of dehydration and malnutrition.

Liver function test: Malnutrition related to eating disorders can cause liver damage.

Measurement of cholesterol: Anorexia or binge disorder can increase blood cholesterol levels.

Thyroid function test: This test controls any problems with the thyroid, which can affect weight. This is an important test for anyone in recovery, which may be able to gain a hard time or lose weight. If necessary, medications will be prescribed for the management of thyroid.

Your health care professional will probably do a thorough analysis of your urine as well. It helps in evaluating kidney function, urine sugar levels, and ketone levels, as it also helps in the diagnosis of systemic diseases and tract disorders. Ketones, which can accumulate within the blood when the body is starved of food and nutrients, indicate that the body is "eating its own fat" for energy. The accumulation of ketones within the blood can lead to ketoacidosis, which can lead to coma and death.

Your health care professional may also take an important sign reading, provide a referral for a bone density test for osteopenia or osteoporosis, and perform an electrocardiogram for heartbeat irregularities.

Chapter 2: Benefits and Disadvantages of Fasting

Main Benefits of Fasting

Weight Loss

In line with a piece of writing published in August 2015 within the Academy of Nutrition and Dietetics Journal, any version of IFT can contribute to weight loss. The researchers examined data from 13 studies and found that the average weight loss for the two-week test ranged from 1.3 percent to eight percent for the two-week trial.

If you are hoping to lose weight, this is probably welcome news. Still, the short-term in those studies means that it is unclear if it is sustainable, and at the end of the day, the extra pounds Can help you keep it closed.

The other catch: the amount of lost weight does not seem to be longer than what you would expect from any other calorie-restricted diet, and by counting the percentage of calories you are eating per day, you will find yourself beneficial. Weight. After all, the diet does not restrict high-calorie foods.

Less important signs may help if less high vital signs within the short term. A study published in June 2018 in Nutrition and Healthy Aging found that 16: 8 participants reduced systolic vital signs in 23 study participants. The link has been shown in both animal and human studies, consistent with a review published in March 2019 in Nutrients. And, an October 2019 study published within the European Journal of Nutrition found that there was an even greater reduction in systolic vital signs compared to another diet in which eating time was not defined.

It is important to have a healthy, vital sign. In essence, unhealthy levels can increase your risk for heart conditions, stroke, and renal disorder.

But research thus far suggests that these vital signs occur only during the practice of IF. Once the diet ended, and others returned to eating normally, researchers found that vital sign readings returned to their initial levels.

Reduces Inflammation

Animal studies have shown that both IF and normal calorie restriction can reduce inflammation levels. However, clinical trials are few and very few. The of a study published in Nutrition Research wanted to understand whether this link also existed among humans. The study included 50 participants, who were fasting for Ramadan, the Muslim holiday, which includes fasting from sunrise to sunset, and eating overnight. The study showed that in the fasting period, pro-inflammatory markers were lower than normal, as were vital signs, weight, and body fat.

Lower Cholesterol

According to a three-week-long study published in Obesity, alternate-day fasting can also help lower total cholesterol in the form of LDL cholesterol when erased in combination with alternative exercise. LDL cholesterol is "bad" cholesterol that will increase the risk of heart disease or stroke, consistent with the Centers for Disease Control and Prevention. Obesity researchers also noted that if the presence of triglycerides is reduced, which are fats found within the blood that would be the cause of a stroke, attack, or heart condition, consistent with the Mayo Clinic. One caveat here: the study was small, so more research is needed to find out if results on cholesterol are long-lasting.

Healthy cholesterol levels and less significant signs (the two benefits above) play a serious role in helping reduce your risk of stroke. But this is not the only possible stroke-related benefit of IF. A piece of writing in Experimental and Translational Stroke Medicine found that a reduction in IF and calories may provide a protective mechanism for the brain in general. In cases where there is a stroke, it seems that eating this way can relieve brain injury. Researchers say that future studies need to find out if a stroke can aid recovery after IF.

Boosted Brain Function

Dr. Gottfried states that IF can improve mental acuity and concentration. And there is some preliminary research to support that idea: A study on mice published in February 2018 in Experimental Biology and Medicine found that it is supposed to help protect against the decline in memory that comes with age. In line with the Johns Hopkins Health Review, IF can improve connections within the hippocampus of the brain and protect against amyloid plaques, which are found in patients with Alzheimer's. This study was only performed in animals; however, it is still unclear whether this benefit is true for humans.

Cancer Protection

Some studies have shown that alternate-day fasting can reduce cancer risk by limiting the occurrence of lymphoma, limiting tumor survival and slowing the proliferation of cancer cells, American Journal of Clinical Consistent with the review of published studies within Nutrition. Studies showing the benefits of cancer were all animal studies; however, more studies are needed to validate an advantage for humans and to understand the mechanisms behind these effects.

Increased Cell Turnover

Gottfried states that the amount of rest involved in intermittent fasting increases autophagy, which is "an important detoxification function within the body to wash away damaged cells." In other words, eating and digestion allow the body to heal and get coarse junk inside cells that will accelerate aging, she says.

A study published in May 2019 in Nutrients found that time-restricted feeding, which researchers defined as eating between 8 am and 1 pm, increased the expression of the autophagy gene LC3A and, therefore, the protein mTOR, which controls cell growth. The study was small, involving only 11 participants for four days. Another study, published in Autophagy in August 2019, also stated that food restriction might be well recognized for increased autophagy, particularly neuronal autophagy, which may provide protective benefits for the brain. There are also some limitations with this study; however: This was done on mice and not on humans.

Low Insulin Resistance

Gottfried proposes that intermittent fasting may help stabilize blood sugar levels in people with diabetes as it resets insulin, although more research is needed.

It has been thought that limiting calories may improve insulin resistance, which may be a marker of type 2 diabetes, consistent with a study published in April 2019 in Nutrients. Fasting, like the type of IF-related fasting, encourages insulin levels to fall, which may play a function to reduce the risk for type 2, the study notes. "I have colleagues from other facilities who have seen positive results in improving insulin needs, especially for diabetic patients," Laudon says.

The above study, published in Nutrition and Healthy Aging, investigated this effect in humans, and while the 16: 8 approach eliminated insulin resistance reduction, the results were not significantly different from the control group. And again, this study was small.

Registered dietitians recommend intermittent fasting to people with diabetes with caution. People on certain medications or insulin for type 2 diabetes (whether managing blood glucose for type 2 or type 1 diabetes) may be at greater risk for low blood sugar, which can be life-threatening. Before trying intermittent fasting, ask your doctor if you have any type of diabetes, they recommend.

Reduced risk of cardiovascular issues

There is a risk of dangerous cardiovascular events when insulin levels fall, such as congestive coronary failure, which is important for patients with type 2 diabetes as opposed to the above nutrients. More likely to die. Heart conditions, compared to adults without diabetes, are consistent with the American Heart Association.

Nutritional studies state that there are no human studies to validate benefits. Still, observational studies have shown whether there can be both cardiovascular and metabolic benefits. The low level of suspicion that changed in metabolic parameters, low levels of triglycerides and decreased blood sugar levels are the results of weight loss and regardless of whether the load was lost, regardless of IF Examples of through a medium or low-carb diet increased longevity are a pair of animal and rodent studies that have shown whether IF can extend lifespan Is, possibly because fasting creates resistance to age-related diseases. A review published in the Current Obesity Report in June 2019 states that while these findings are promising, they are difficult to replicate in human studies. Until this happens, it is best to doubt about this potential benefit.

A better night's sleep

If you've ever felt like you've slipped into a food coma after a huge meal, you believe that the diet can influence waking up and falling asleep. Some IF followers report better sleeping ability as a result of following this method of eating. "If sleep can affect food and food," says Rose-Francis. Why?

One theory is that IF regulates biological time, which determines sleep patterns. A regulated biological time means that you can easily stop research and feel refreshed to support this theory, however, in line with a piece of writing published in December 2018 in Sleep of Nature and Science.

The second principle centers on the fact that having a meal first in the evening means that you will digest the food until you hit the pillow. In line with the National Sleep Foundation, digestion is complete when you are upright, and a full stomach roll may cause acid reflux or heartburn at bedtime, making it difficult to stop.

People prefer to fast for many reasons, whether they are related to health, weight loss, finances, or religion. Fasting can only range from juice-fasting to fasting that excludes all food and liquids, such as dry fasting. While fasting can sometimes bring some health benefits, they can also be very dangerous. Fasting hurts the short and future and has a detrimental effect on many people, including those they want to reduce. Ultimately, the consequences of avoiding food differ substantially from that of a fasting person.

Weight management fasting can be detrimental to weight management, which is consistent with dietitians registered on mayoclinic.com. After a period of fasting, research shows that people crave starchy foods with high-calorie content. Carbohydrates are the body's favorite source of fuel. Excessive hunger also causes you to get more calories, which is healthy for the body to consume in one sitting. Finally, fasting can reverse the intended effects of a weight management plan.

Short-term side effects term side effects, the Fasting has several short-American Cancer Society reports. These include headache, dizziness, lighthouse, fatigue, low vital signs, and abnormal heart rhythm. Fasting people may experience an impaired ability to perform certain tasks, such as operating machinery or driving vehicles. Fasting can also lead to some conditions such as gout or gallstones. Fasting may impair the body's ability to absorb certain medications, or there may be changes in drug interactions within the body.

Long-Term Side Effects

Fasting also has harmful effects in the future. Not only can fasting damage the system, but it can also negatively affect many parts of the body, including the liver and kidneys. Fasting can interfere with important bodily processes. For example, avoiding eating in already malnourished people can be dangerous. It is also possible to fast at the time of death when the accumulated energy of the body is completely exhausted.

Dry fasting is one of the worst mistakes to avoid when trying to lose weight, in fact, it reduces the consumption of all fluids and liquid food, and is particularly dangerous.

Dry fasting can quickly lead to dehydration and death in only a few days. The American Cancer Society reported that the health effects of fasting vary substantially by person and context. Factors such as heat, heavy labor, and compromised health can make dry fasting fatal in just a few hours.

Chapter 3: Advantages of Intermittent Fasting

When you don't eat for a short time, there are many things that change in your body:

For example, your body initiates important cellular repair processes and changes hormone levels to make stored body fat more accessible.

Main Body Changes

Here are several changes that occur in your body during fasting:

- *Insulin Levels*: Insulin blood levels are significantly reduced, which facilitates fat burning.
- Human Somatotropin: The maximum amount of blood in the growth hormone can increase up to 5 times. High levels of this hormone provide fat burning and muscle gain and have many other benefits.
- Cellular Repair: The body induces important cellular repair processes, such as the removal of waste from cells.

- Gene Expression: Many genes and molecules associated with longevity and protection from disease undergo beneficial changes.

Intermittent fasting can help you lose weight and belly fat, many of which try to stop intermittently, to reduce it. Generally, intermittent fasting will cause you to eat less food. Unless you compensate by eating more during the opposite meal, you will find yourself consuming fewer calories. Additionally, intermittent fasting increases hormone function to facilitate weight loss. Low insulin levels, high somatotropin levels, and increased amounts of norepinephrine (noradrenaline) all increase the breakdown of body fat and facilitate energy use.

For this reason, short-term fasting increases your rate by 3.6–14%, helping you burn even more calories. In other words, intermittent fasting works on each side of the calorie equation. It increases your rate (increases calories) and reduces the amount of food you eat (reduces calories). Intermittent fasting can reduce weight by 3–8% in 3–24 weeks, consistent with a 2014 review of the scientific literature. This is often a large amount.

People lost 4-7% of their waist circumference, indicating they had lost abdominal fat, the harmful fat inside the abdomen that causes disease. A review study also showed that intermittent fasting caused less muscle loss than sustained caloric restriction. Intermittent fasting can reduce insulin resistance, reducing your risk of type 2 diabetes has become incredibly common in recent decades.

Its main feature is high blood sugar levels in the context of insulin resistance. Anything that reduces insulin resistance should help lower blood sugar levels and protect against type 2 diabetes. Interestingly, intermittent fasting is of major benefit for insulin resistance and causes a powerful decrease in blood sugar levels. In human studies on intermittent fasting, fasting blood glucose is reduced by 3–6%, while fasting insulin is reduced by 20–31%. A study in diabetic mice has also shown that intermittent fasting is protected against kidney damage, which is one of the serious complications of diabetes. What this suggests is that intermittent fasting may be highly protective for those at risk of developing type 2 diabetes.

Benefits of Intermittent Fasting

Intermittent fasting can reduce oxidative stress and inflammation in the body. Oxidative stress is one of many stages of aging and chronic diseases. It contains unstable molecules called free radicals, which react with and damage other important molecules (such as proteins and DNA). Several studies suggest that intermittent fasting may increase the body's resistance to oxidative stress. Additionally, studies suggest that intermittent fasting may help fight inflammation, another major driver of all types of common diseases.

Intermittent fasting can also be beneficial for heart health, that is currently the world's largest killer.

It is known that various health markers (so-called "risk factors") are related to an increased or decreased risk of a heart condition. Intermittent fasting has been shown to increase many different risk factors, including vital signs, total and LDL cholesterol, blood triglycerides, inflammatory markers, and blood sugar levels. However, the cargo of this is often supported by animal studies. Consequences on heart health are studied for tonsils occurring in humans; recommendations are often made.

Intermittent fasting indicates various cellular repair processes.

When we fast, the cells within the body initiate an auto play "waste removal" process known as autophagy. It involves breaking and metabolizing the broken and lax proteins that build up inside cells over time. Increased autophagy may protect against many diseases, including cancer and Alzheimer's disease.

Intermittent fasting can help prevent cancer. It can be a terrible disease, characterized by the uncontrolled growth of cells. Fasting has been shown to have several beneficial effects on metabolism, which will reduce the risk of cancer. Although human studies are needed, evidence from animal studies indicates that intermittent fasting may help prevent cancer. There is also some evidence on human cancer patients, showing that fasting reduced the various side effects of chemotherapy.

Intermittent fasting is sweet for your brain, which is good for the body; it is also generally good for the brain. Intermittent fasting improves various metabolic characteristics important for brain health. This includes reduced oxidative stress, reduced inflammation, and blood sugar levels, and relaxation of insulin resistance. Several studies in mice have shown that intermittent fasting can increase the expansion of the latest nerve cells, which should have benefits for brain function. It also increases levels of a brain hormone called brain-derived neurotrophic factor (BDNF), a deficiency of which has been implicated in depression and various other brain problems. Animal studies have also shown that intermittent fasting protects against brain damage.

Intermittent fasting can help prevent Alzheimer's disease. Alzheimer's disease is the world's most common neurodegenerative disease. There is no cure available for Alzheimer's, so it is important to avoid exposure in the first place.

A study in mice suggests that intermittent fasting may delay the onset of Alzheimer's disease or reduce its severity. During a series of case reports, a lifestyle intervention that included daily short-term fasting was set to significantly improve Alzheimer's symptoms in 9 out of 10 patients. Animal studies also suggest that fasting can protect against other neurodegenerative diseases, including Parkinson's and Huntington's course.

Intermittent fasting can increase your lifespan, helping you live longer. One of the most exciting applications of intermittent fasting may also be its ability to extend lifespan.

Studies conducted in mice have shown that intermittent fasting extends lifespan during sustained caloric restriction in a similar manner. In a number of these studies, the results were quite dramatic. In one of them, mice fasting every other day lived 83% longer than mice, not fasting. Although it is often far from proven in humans, intermittent fasting has become very fashionable among the anti-aging crowd. Given the known benefits for metabolism and each type of health marker, it is sensible that intermittent fasting can help you live an extended and healthy life.

Chapter 4: The Self-Cleaning Process of Autophagy

Maybe a cellular pathway involved in autophagy, or cellular self-digestion, protein and organelle degradation, surprising the connection to human disease with number and physiology. For example, autophagic dysfunction is related to cancer, neurodegeneration, microbial infections, and aging. Paradoxically, although autophagy is primarily a protective process for the cell, it may also play a function in necrobiosis. Understanding autonomy may eventually allow scientists and practitioners to use this process to improve human health.

At first glance, it seems surprising that the process of cellular self-feeding can be beneficial. In its simplest form, however, autophagy probably represents a cell's adaptation to starvation. If no food is available within the environment, a cell is forced to disrupt a part of its reserves until those things don't get better. In single-cell organisms such as yeast, this starvation response is one of the first functions of autophagy. Still, this role extends through humans. For example, even on a day-to-day basis, autophagy is activated between meals, supplying amino acids and energy through catabolism to organs such as the liver to take care of their metabolic functions.

Different Types of Autophagy

There are various types of autophagy, including micro-macroautophagic, also in the form of chaperone-mediated autophagy (CMA), and they differ in their mechanisms and functions. Both micro- and macroautophagic can attach large structures through both selective and non-selective mechanisms. At the same time, CMA only decays soluble proteins, albeit selectively. The ability to mass degrade autophagic function is important. Still, it carries a special risk, as uncontrolled degradation of the cytoplasm is probably going to be fatal.

On the other hand, the basal level of autophagy is important for maintaining normal cellular homeostasis. Thus, it is important that the autophagy is tightly regulated so that it is induced when necessary, but otherwise maintained at a basal level. Although a complete picture of autophagy regulation is not available, recent reviews cover several aspects.

The survival function of autophagy has been demonstrated at the cell and organism levels in many contexts, including nutritional and protein deficiencies, endoplasmic reticulum stress, development, microbial infection, and diseases characterized by the formation of protein aggregation. This survival-protecting function is generally considered adaptive, but, in the context of cancer, potentially fatal. Metabolic stress can be a common feature of the tumor microenvironment, and most chemotherapeutic agents induce cellular stress. Thus, there is a neighborhood of intensive scrutiny as to whether autophagy-dependent survival should be inhibited in these settings to market tumor-cell death.

A clear relationship is that autophagy functions in both cytoprotecting and necrobiosis. In response to most types of cellular stress, autophagy plays a cytoprotective role, as ATG gene knockdown/knockout accelerates rather than delayed necrobiosis. However, in some settings where there is an uncontrolled reduction of autophagy (egg, overplant 1 of the autophagy protein in mammalian cells, and Atg1 overgrowth in Drosophila 15), autophagy can cause necrobiosis, possibly as a result of apoptosis or possibly as a result of activating. To avoid nonspecific degradation of cytoplasmic material in massive amounts of cells. Many samples of ATG-gene dependent necrobiosis are caused by a lack of cells in apoptosis, suggesting that autophagy, as a pathway to necrobiosis, may also be an alternative to pus Aller. A general caveat for those types of studies is that overexpression or knockout of an ATG gene may have unknown indirect effects beyond autophagy.

Autophagic programmed necrobiosis was originally described in tissues undergoing active development. Nevertheless, not only is there no evidence that ATG gene inhibition prevents this death, but the other may also be true. Nematodes are lacking bec-1, Caenorhabditis orthologs of ATG6 / Belin, and mice lacking Belin 1 or atg5 display increased numbers of apoptotic cells in fetal tissue, which is autophagic in developmentally sorted necrobiosis. It is against the need for machinery. However, it may be premature to conclude that autophagy deficiency leads to increased generation of apoptotic cells during development, as the ATG machinery also plays a role within the removal of apoptotic corpses. In mature animals with tissue-specific

ATG gene knockout, there is clear evidence of the anti-apoptotic function of autopsy in vivo.

Crosstalk between autophagy, a pathway that functions predominantly in cell survival, and apoptosis, a pathway that always results in necrobiosis, is complex. Common factors regulate the two pathways; they share common components and can regulate and modify the activity of each opposite. Many of the signals originally studied in the context of apoptosis activation induce autophagy. At the same time, signals that prevent apoptosis also inhibit autophagy. Anti-apoptotic proteins, such as the Bcl-2 affinity, inhibit Belin, and pro-apoptotic factors such as BH-only proteins, inhibit this inhibitory interaction and thereby activate autophagy.

Another link between the autophagic machinery and apoptosis is that Atg5 that can undergo a calpain-mediated cleavage to obtain a pro-apoptotic fragment that functions within the inner mitochondrial death pathway. These examples can only represent the tip of the iceberg, as we are just beginning to understand the complex molecular differences between autophagy and apoptosis. However, it seems likely that the coordinated regulation of 'self-digestion' by autophagy and 'self-killing' by apoptosis may underlie various aspects of growth, tissue homeostasis, and disease pathogenesis.

Neurodegeneration evidence of growth suggests that changes in autophagy occur in many human diseases. Here we discuss only those disorders during which autophagy dysfunction has been shown to contribute to their pathogenesis. As noted above, autophagy occurs at basal, constitutive levels, and studies to date have highlighted the importance of basal autophagy in internal intracellular control. Basal autophagy demand varies across tissues; This is particularly important within the liver and in other tissues, where cells, such as neurons and myocytes, do not divide after differentiation.

In contrast to standard atg5, atgatg5, and Belin 1 knockout mice, those who die during embryogenesis or neonatal period 1 survive a period of postnatal starvation after nerve-tissue-specific knockout of those genes. However, these mice develop progressive motor deficits and exhibit abnormal reflexes, and ubiquitin-positive inclusion bodies accumulate in their neurons. Although the amount of autophagosomes found in neurons is very low in normal and even starvation conditions, these studies demonstrate that the constitutional turnover of cytosolic content by autophagy is associated with any disease-related mutant. It is also unavoidable in the absence of protein expression.

Despite the important function of basal autophagy in healthy individuals, the need for autophagy under disease conditions is even more pronounced. Recent studies suggest that erosion of disease-related mutant proteins is very much associated with autophagy, in addition to the ubiquitin-proteasome system. Examples include extended polyglutamine-containing proteins that cause various neurodegenerative diseases such as Huntington's disease and spinocerebellar ataxia and mutant types of α-synuclein that cause familial Parkinson's disease. CMA also participates in wild-type α-synuclein degradation, but the mutant type of α-synuclein blocks the lysosomal receptor, leading to normal CMA inhibition. Affected cells plan to capture CMA by upgrading macroautophagic to catch the blockage, which guarantees cell survival but makes cells more susceptible to stresses.

Considering all the available data, there is little question that autophagy is a beneficial effect of protecting against neurodegeneration; However, how autism can prevent neurodegeneration is not fully understood. One hypothesis is that autophagy terminates protein aggregates or inclusion bodies, possibly in a directed manner. One possible adapter is p62 / sequestosome-1 (SQSTM1). Most protein aggregates are decorated with ubiquitin, and SQSTM1 contains both LC3-binding (the mammalian homolog of the autophagy-related protein Atg8) and ubiquitin-binding domains, considering the popularity of protein aggregates by a protein within it (LC3) Huh. Autophagosome-forming membrane. Also, proper trading of p62 by autofellatio is important to prevent spontaneous aggregation formation.

However, the direct degradation of aggregates by autophagy is somehow contradictory to the recent hypothesis that the generation of protein aggregates may be a protective mechanism. Rather, the first target of autophagy is the spreading cytosolic protein, not the inclusion of the body itself, suggesting that cellular inclusion in autophagy-deficient cells is an opportunity for impaired normal protein turnover. However, it is still possible that misfolded proteins insoluble or oligomeric states may be preferentially recognized by autophagosome membranes, which may also be mediated by the ubiquitin – p62 – LC3 interactions.

Alzheimer's changes have also been observed in Alzheimer's disease. Still, during this case, the contribution of hoarseness may not be as simple as other types of neurodegeneration. For example, autophagosome-like structures accumulate in dystrophic neurites and model mice of Alzheimer's disease, possibly in autolysosomes due to lack of maturation of autophagosomes. Surprisingly, toxic proteolytic products A often originates within these partially degraded compartments because the A protein precursor protein, APP, and, therefore, the protease responsible for its cleavage are both present within the sequential endoplasmic reticulum in these structures. Therefore, one hypothesis is that impaired autophagic flow provides a unique site for Aβ peptide production.

It is reasonable to assume that autophagy due to its protective role, maybe a therapeutic target for the treatment of those neurodegenerative diseases. For example, the regulatory protein kinase complex of rapamycin and its corresponding CCI-779-like rapamycin (TOR) inhibitors prevents the degradation of autophagy by the target of rapamycin (TOR) inhibitors from the neurodegeneration observed in the polyglutamine model in Drosophila and mice.

Recently, small-molecule enhancers of rapamycin were identified. These mutants improve the clearance of haunting in and α-synuclein and protect against neurodegeneration during a fruit-fly Huntington's disease model. Importantly, the results of small-molecule enhancers of rapamycin are independent of TOR, making it possible to use them with rapamycin for therapeutic purposes. However, in an attempt to clinically manipulate autophagy, it is necessary to consider the dynamic nature of changes occurring within the autophagic system during the pathological course of the disease.

The innate and adaptive immune disposal of intracellular organisms, almost like cellular organisms, represents a steric challenge to degenerative cellular pathways that would typically be met by autopsy. Equivalent autophagic machinery to selectively capture cellular organelles is employed for selective delivery of microorganisms to lysosomes during a process called habitual xenophagy46. In mammals (and perhaps other metazoan organisms), the role of autophagy in antimicrobial defense probably extends beyond the direct elimination of pathogens. An increasing number of studies indicate a function for autophagy in the delivery of microbial antigenic material to the innate and adaptive system, as well as in maintaining lymphocyte homeostasis 47,48.

Xerophagy can target unicellular bacteria that invade bacteria and parasites residing within the vacuole containing cytosol, phagosomes, or pathogens, also as newly synthesized viruses during their exit from the nucleus via the cytoplasm 47,49. The cell biology of xerophagy is a small amount of well-studied compared to classical autophagy. Despite the overlap in the molecular components required for the two processes, it is not yet clear whether membranes associated with microorganisms have a similar or There are different classical autophagosomes. Pathogen-containing LC3-positive compartments are often much larger than the classical autophagosome, specifically containing the cellular component, indicating plasticity of the autophagic process that allows it to adapt to the need to attach microorganisms. Which are larger than their organisms, an ability that reflects unique mechanisms of autophagosome formation. Although xerophagy appears to be primarily a selective type of autophagy, almost nothing is understood as to how the autophagic machinery recognizes microbes (or membranes containing microbes).

Beyond its direct role in pathogen elimination, autophagy may enhance cytoprotective functions in infected cells and mediate trafficking events required for innate and adaptive immunity. In the case of some RNA viral infections, viral nucleic acids require autophagy for activation of the endosomal toll-like receptor TLR7, and later type I interferon cajoling 47. The autophagic machinery is primarily used for the presentation of histocompatibility complex (MHC) class II, which is the presentation of some endogenously synthesized viral antigen 47. Not only does the autophagic machinery function in innate and adaptive immunity, but many innate and adaptive immune mediators are involved in intracellular pathogen control that stimulates autophagia 47.

Given the different roles of hoarseness in innate and adaptive immunity, it is not surprising that many pathogens have devised strategies to exclude hoarseness. Some intracellular bacteria and viruses co-opt the autophagic machinery to use Ag protein-dependent dynamic membrane rearrangements at their own repulsive benefits

49,50. More commonly, successful intracellular pathogens regulate signaling pathways that regulate autophagy or block the events of membranous trafficking required for autophagy-mediated pathogen delivery to lysosome 47. In some settings, microbial evasion of autophagy may also be necessary for microbial pathogenesis. For example, lethal herpes simplex virus encephalitis requires inhibition of berlin one autophagy protein by the pandemic neurovirulence protein 51. Thus, selective disruption of interactions between microbial virulence factors and their target host cytosis proteins may help reduce infection-induced morbidity.

Other postulated roles of autophagy in immunity that receive further scientific attention include T-cell homeostasis, central and peripheral tolerance induction, and, therefore the prevention of unwanted inflammation and autoimmunity 47. We also note that several recent genome-wide scans have revealed strong associations between a non-synonymous single nucleotide polymorphism within the autophagy gene ATG16L1, also within the autonomy-stimulating immune-related GTPase IRGM, and for Crohn's disease. As a sensitivity. intestine13. These associations suggest an intriguing potential role for autophagy deregulation within the pathogenesis of Crohn's disease. However, it is not known whether the ATG16L variant is defective in autophagy function and whether this genetic association is indicative of a mechanistic link between autophagy impairment and Crohn's disease pathogenesis. Studies in targeted mutant mice with the knock-in T300A mutation in ATG16L1 will help clarify these important questions.

Over the past decade, there has been an incredible advancement in our knowledge about the molecular mechanisms of macro autophagy, including the identification of several components of the protein mechanism. By comparison, our understanding of regulation, particularly the complex interactions of multiple stimulatory and inhibitory inputs, is comparatively limited. Given its dual capacity to control autophagy for therapeutic purposes, especially in cytoprotecting and necrobiosis, we would like to increase our understanding of various regulatory pathways.

Our understanding of other types of autophagy is limited, in contrast to the rapid advances within the molecular dissection of macro autophagy and the increasing information about its regulation and its pathophysiological relevance. Important molecular players for CMA are identified, but other regulatory components remain to be discovered, by comparison with other membrane translation systems. Currently, available information about microphage is even more limited, and therefore the absence of reliable markers or assays to detect this process has prevented any connection of macroautophagic changes with physiological or pathological conditions.

Although adaptation to starvation or stress is a conserved function of the development of hoarseness under physiological conditions, erosion of intracellular components may also be a more important function when considering the role of autophagy in disease. An area of future interest is to review how autophagy acts to prevent neurodegeneration.

However, we do not currently know direct details for the toxicity of neuropeptides such as Au and α-synuclein. Additionally, we would like to know the difficulty of functional autophagy playing a protective role, as opposed to compromised autophagy and therefore with the accumulation of cytosolic autophagosomes, which in these latter conditions neurologic, disease, and myopathy Contributes to pathogenesis, as autophagy contributes to these latter conditions can increase disease pathology. Similarly, we should always carefully consider whether autophagy inhibition or exacerbation is probably going to be beneficial when progressing diseases such as cancer and when attempting to work out. To better understand immunity, it will be important to spot the mechanisms by which autophagy is activated in response to microbial invasion, targets that allow specific identification of intracellular pathogens, and, therefore, in immune system function. Role of autophagy.

One of the current challenges within the study of autophagy in old age is that most of the genetic mouse models with impaired autophagy do not reproduce most features of aging-dependent changes. These models have complete obstruction of autophagy and this obstruction is present from birth. The recent introduction of conditional knockout mice should partially help to defeat this problem, as they make it possible to match the consequences of impaired autophagy at birth when compensatory mechanisms are likely to be activated within adulthood. Occurrence

Thus, although tremendous progress has been made in our understanding of autophagy, many unanswered questions remain. A full understanding of all types of autophagy is necessary before we can expect to control these pathways for the treatment of human disease.

Autophagy means "self-eating" - but rest assured, it is often an honest thing. Autophagy is the method by which your body cleans up damaged cells and toxins, helping you to regenerate new, healthy cells.

Over time, our cells accumulate the proliferation of dead organisms, damaged proteins and oxidized particles that inhibit the internal functioning of the body. This accelerates the consequences of aging and age-related diseases because cells are not normally divided and ready to perform.

Since many of our cells, such as those within the brain, get to last a lifetime, the body developed a unique way to distance itself from these defective parts and naturally defend against disease. Enter: Autophagy.

How Does Autophagy Process Work?

Think of your body as a kitchen, after preparing the meal, clean the counter, pack and recycle the leftovers. Then you'll have a clean kitchen and can reuse the stored food later. This is what happens automatically in our body with the self-cleaning process of Autophagy.

Now, consider a similar scenario, but you are older and not efficient. After making your meal, you allow the residue on the counter. It has several rubbishes; its number does not. Swinging pieces on counters, litter, and bin. They don't make it out the door to a dumpster, and toxic industrial waste starts to build in your kitchen. There is food fermentation on the ground, and every kind of filthy smell comes out of the door.

Due to the onslaught of pollutants and toxins, you must maintain a hard time with daily grinding. This scenario resembles autophagy, which is not working as it should be.

Autophagy typically moves silently behind the scenes in maintenance mode. It plays a function within the way your body reacts in times of stress, maintaining balance and controlling cellular function.

There is evidence that once you trigger autophagy, you interrupt the aging process, reduce inflammation and boost your overall performance. To resist your body's illness and support longevity, you will naturally increase your vocal response.

Humanity and longevity evolved from long-term physical activity to famine, our ability to respond to biological stresses over a long period. A study at the University of Newcastle found that this ability is thanks to small adaptations during a protein referred to as p62 that induces autophagy.

By sensing metabolic byproducts that cause cell damage (called reactive oxygen species ROS), protein p62 activates autophagy or initiates cleaning. P62 protein removes all damaged items stored in your body so that you are better equipped to deal with biological stress. Homeostasis (balanced cellular function) and vibrant health are the immediate results of the p62 protein doing its thing during autophagy. As a result, damaged goods that build up in your body over time become a brand new to cell formation - and this is the thing that keeps you healthy.

While humans possess this ability, instead some lower creatures like for example flies don't have. Therefore, the research team set about identifying a portion of the human protein p62 that allows for the sensing of ROS. They then produced genetically modified flies with "humanized" p62.

Result? "Humanized" flies live longer under stressful conditions.

This shows us that capabilities such as sensing stress and activating protective processes such as autophagy can develop to allow for better stress resistance and an extended life span.

Advantages of Autophagy

We are only beginning to understand how this works within the body, and we all know that this type is still based on rodent studies. Mice are not men, but the evidence is compelling

- Money control inflammation, interfere with the process of aging and neurodegenerative protect against Rogue
- may help fight infections and support immune
- triggers can be Bhoomika support increased kite long
- how to autophagy
- There are ways to cause the melancholy process of your body (that there is nothing to try to clear the juice). To cleanse your cells and reduce inflammation, and generally keep your body running in tip-top shape, follow these five simple steps to expand the autophagy process.

Keep in mind that since dreaming can be a reaction to anxiety, you might want to trick your body into thinking it is a touch bit. Here's how:

1. Eat a high-fat, low-carb

emphasizes the importance of eating fat to activate. "Fat should be the major macronutrient in our diet because it is different from protein. While protein can become a car and sugar, [not fat]," she says.

2. Continue a protein fast.

Once or twice a week, limit your protein consumption to 15-25 grams each day. This provides your body with a full day to recycle protein, which can help reduce inflammation and cleanse your cells without any muscle loss. During this point, while autophagy is triggered, your body is forced to consume its proteins and toxins.

3. Practice Intermittent

Autophagy Fasting Research shows that fasting increases. How long for autophagy? During a 2010 study, mice fasted for twenty-four or 48 hours to bring autophagy to market. It is unclear how this translates into humans (yet). Still, we know that intermittent fasting is related to weight loss, insulin sensitivity, and reduced disease risk.

4. Exercise

Another reason to hit the gym: In human and rodent studies, exercise has been shown to stimulate autophagy. During a 2018 study, 12 men completed an eight-week exercise program, including continuous state cycling or high-intensity interval cycling for up to 3 days per week. The researchers concluded that both types of training supported autophagy, which supports the idea that every single movement is a sweet movement.

Macro autophagy (autophagy) may be a lysosomal degradation pathway for the breakdown of intracellular proteins and organelles. Although constitutional autophagy may be a homeostatic mechanism for autism recycling and metabolic regulation, autophagy is additionally stressed responsive, where it is important to remove damaged proteins and organelles. Thus, autophagy limits stress tolerance, limits damage and maintain viability under adverse conditions. Autophagy may be a tumor suppression mechanism, yet it enables tumor cell survival under stress. Demonstrating how a prosecutive loss can promote tumorigenesis, emerging evidence suggests that preservation of cellular fitness by autophagy may also be important for tumor suppression. Since autophagy is such a fundamental process that establishes how the functional state of autophagy affects tumorigenicity and the treatment response is important. This is often particularly important as many current cancer physicians activate autophagy. Therefore, efforts to unravel and modify the autophagy pathway will provide new approaches to cancer therapy and prevention.

Autophagy may be a lysosomal degradation pathway for intracellular digestion.

Stress stimuli activate cellular pathways for adaptation that are important for cells to either tolerate unfavorable conditions or to eliminate damaged and potentially dangerous cells. For example, cells like apoptosis trigger suicide mechanisms. Metabolic stress, including starvation, increases the cellular requirement for energy production and damage mitigation and plays an important role in both instances of catabolic cellular self-digestion by autophagy. Stress activates autophagy where double-membrane vesicles are formed and Anglo proteins, cytoplasm, protein aggregates, and organelles are then transported to the lysosome where they are degraded. It acts to take care of cellular metabolism through the recycling of cellular components when the supply of sources of external nutrients is restricted. Autophagy-deficient mice have tissues with low ATP levels and fail to survive the period of neonatal starvation, providing a transparent example of autophagy-mediated management of energy homeostasis. Stress, particularly that resulting from oxidative damage to aging or hypoxic conditions, causes damage to proteins and organelles that require autophagy to eradicate. Mice with autophagy defects accumulate cells with polyubiquitinated, p62 (centrosome 1) - related protein aggregates and damaged mitochondria and show elevated oxidative stress and necrobiosis. Thus, autophagy is important for the degrading turnover of proteins and organisms damaged during stress, the failure of which is toxic to cells and tissues and can be pro-inflammatory. Peptides resulting from proteins degraded by autophagy can also be used in T cells for immune and host defense for antigen presentation. The importance of autophagy as a homeostatic and survival-promoting mechanism is underscored by the association of autophagy defects within the etiology of several diseases, including neurodegeneration, steatosis, regional enteritis, infection, aging, and cancer.

Autophagy emphasizes metabolism in areas with tumors. In normal cells, autophagy is activated in tumor cells by stress, including starvation, hypoxia, and factor deprivation. Tumor cells experience nutrient-enhanced metabolic stress, factors due to insufficient blood supply and oxygen deficiency as a result of deficient angiogenesis. This environmental metabolic stress in tumors is complicated by cell-intrinsic metabolic stress derived from high metabolic demands of cell proliferation and altered metabolism (aerobic glycolysis) where ATP production is impaired. Autophagy localizes to hypoxic areas of the tumor that are farthest to the blood vessels where it supports tumor cell survival. Thus, autophagy plays a similar role in tumor cells as it does in normal cells. Still, because the underlying stress tumor cells face larger, dependence on autophagy may also be more substantial. This distinction between normal and tumor cells in the context of autophagy dependence may also be useful for the exploitation of autophagy modulation in cancer therapy by providing a therapeutic window. Additionally, the tumor mass consists of heterogeneous regions of vessel and nutrient supply, and tumor cells residing in hypoxic tumor areas undergoing autophagy are tumor cells that resist radiation and chemotherapy. Knowing that autophagy supports the survival of this important subfamily of tumor cells provides a chance to focus on these resistant cells to enhance cancer therapy.

Main Benefits of Autophagy

Autophagy promotes the metabolism of tumor cells to metabolic stress. One of the notable functions within the repertoire of tumor cells is to activate autophagy in response to a concern allowing prolonged survival, especially when apoptosis is flawed. Generally, apoptosis will eliminate tumor cells, which eliminate inducible stress as a tumor suppression mechanism. Tumor cells often develop defects in apoptosis, allowing survival to last for weeks in a state of isolation. Tumor cells can progressively eat themselves under prolonged stress, but one-third of their normal size. During the method of cellular consumption via autophagy, cellular division and motility are suppressed which may represent an energy conservation effort. "dormant" tumor cells represent minimal cells capable of recovery (MCCRs), capable of returning to their normal size and resuming cell proliferation within 24 hours of restoring normal growth conditions. She holds. Autophagy should be a highly selective process to allow extensive cellular degradation while maintaining functional integrity. How cellular components are selected and directed to the autophagy pathway for degradation is important. Still, it likely involves specialized processes such as mitophagy and p62 protein aggregate formation. Establishing latency with the potential for regeneration is highly skewed in the autophagy, as tumor cells with autophagy defects are less efficient at reducing and reproducing autoimmunity. Thus, autophagy limits tumor cells with improved stress tolerance that limits damage, maintains viability, maintains dormancy, and facilitates recovery.

A major aspect of cancer treatment is the influx of injury and stress on tumor cells, enough to kill them with an alternative type of apoptosis, necrosis, or necrobiosis. However, a small number of leftover tumor cells are simple enough for the tumor, often years later, with fatal results. The remaining tumor cells that manage to tolerate treatment and persist in re-emerging later point can be a basic barrier to successful cancer treatment. The mechanism by which tumor cells elicit inactivation and regenerate, and therefore the precise role of autophagy in these processes, must be defined. Therapeutic targeting of autophagy for attenuation and regeneration is well worth it. Still, there may also be additional opportunities to target the inactivation and regeneration pathway specifically.

Autophagy is suppressed in many human tumors, although autophagy may be a survival pathway used by both normal and tumor cells to avoid starvation and stress, paradoxically, autophagy defects are found in many human tumors Huh. Alkaline loss of the essential autophagy gene dblin1 often occurs in human breast, ovarian, and prostate cancers. This limited evaluation requires further confirmation with the evaluation of other autophagy genes coupled with the functional analysis of autophagy in tumors. Alkaline loss of Beclin1 also presents to mice susceptible to hepatoma (HCC), lung adenocarcinoma, breast hyperplasia, and lymphoma. Deficiency within defective autophagy or the essential autophagy gene atg5 through the defective loss of Belin 1 promotes tumorigenesis of immortal epithelial kidneys and mammary cell lines. Loss of other autophagy regulators such as bif-1 and atg4C also risks mice tumors. However, constitutional activation of the PI-3 kinase pathway may also occur, although the most common mutational event affecting tone is in tumors.

Mammalian targets of PI-3 kinase and rapamycin (mTOR) activation are among the most common events in human cancer, and mTOR inhibits autophagy. The PI-3 kinase pathway serves to integrate protein and nutrient availability with biosynthetic processes such as protein translation and anabolic metabolism in favor of cell growth and proliferation. This allows cells to manage activity and metabolic demand with a supply of external nutrients supplied. When nutrients and growth factors are readily available, the demand for autophagy's catabolic activity is reduced by mTOR.

Under starvation conditions, the PI-3 kinase pathway and the activity of mTOR are suppressed, which regulate cellular biosynthetic processes and cellular proliferation, but de-represses autophagy to enable catabolism. This allows cells to adapt to environmental fluctuations by adjusting behavior, usage, and consumption. This case arises in cancer cells where the PI-3 kinase pathway is constitutively activated by mutation. This causes cell growth signals unrelated to nutrient and protein availability. While signs of constitutional growth drive tumor cell proliferation, it also prepares to reduce tumor cells to induce autophagy or suppress consumption in response to anxiety leading to metabolic catastrophe, where energetic demand exceeds production. This metabolic fragility of tumor cells suggests therapeutic starvation as an approach to cancer therapy to take advantage of the inherent differences between normal and tumor cells. Collectively these findings suggest that although autophagy supports tumor cell survival, many tumors can paradoxically suppress autophagy. In the case of constitutive activation of the PI-3 kinase pathway, the benefit of controlling cell growth may outweigh the survival losses conferred by suppressed autophagy. Alternatively, there may also be additional aspects of autoimmune defects that promote oncogenesis that hold a survival deficit.

The physiological context of autophagy in cancer

A remaining question is whether the role autophagy plays in oncogene activation and tumor suppressor inactivation is like the stress that would increase the need for autophagy. Hypoxia induces hypoxia-inducible transcription factor 1α (Hif-1α), which activates autophagy as a part of a stress-responsive and adaptive transcription program that also promotes angiogenesis and Aβ metabolism.

Induction of Hif-1α for inactivation of von Hippel-Lindau (VHDL) tumor suppressor proteins occurs at high frequency in renal clear cell carcinoma. Still, the contribution of autoimmunity during this setting is known. Loss of retinoblastoma (RB) tumor suppressor protein represses the HIF-1α target Bnip3 and promotes autophagy and necrobiosis. This means that autophagy can protect from RB inactivation by enabling cellular protection. Loss of checkpoint regulation may also increase tumor cell damage that would be countered by autophagy-mediated proteins and organelle internal control monitoring to limit tumor progression. P53 deficiency or mutation within the tumor sphincter promotes autophagy. This p53 may flow from the debris generated by the loss of the DNA damage checkpoint, or the mechanism has not yet been determined. Induction of indomitable type p53 also activates autophagy that would flow from direct transcriptional activation of down-pro-autophagy regulators such as DRAM or perhaps p53 is an indirect result of modulating cellular metabolism. p19Arf induces autophagy and necrobiosis, a small mitochondrial type of tumor suppression, but whether it is often associated with Art tumor suppression is not clear. Finally, the endoplasmic reticulum interacts with Bcl-2 with Belin 1 and suppresses autopsy; However, starvation disrupts this interaction, requiring autophagy to be replaced. Bcl-2 inhibits apoptosis and promotes tumorigenesis in autophagy-deficient cells as well, suggesting that suppression of autophagy by Bcl-2 is not an important factor controlling tumorigenesis. Thus, the role of autophagy in cancer should be evaluated in the context of genetic makeup and the environment of the tumor. Therefore, the guiding principles here are currently lacking.

Autophagy limits necrobiosis and inflammation

One consequence of autophagy defects in tumors is impaired stress, which culminates in chronic tumor necrobiosis. Superficially, stimulation of necrobiosis in tumors may be a desirable outcome. However, persistent chronic necrobiosis stimulates an inflammatory response that will be pro-tumorigenic (36). Dead cells, particularly apoptosis-defective cells that undergo necrotic necrobiosis, which releases cellular material, potentially activate a pro-inflammatory immune response. Nuclear protein is released from high mobility group protein B1 (HMG1) necrotic cells, where it is a ligand for the cell surface receptor for advanced glycation end products (RAGE), which is a potent catalyst for NF-dB.

Similarly, nucleic acids released from necrotic cells can stimulate inflammation through the activation of Toll-like receptors. The presence of molecular patterns (DAMPs) associated with those damage indicates tissue damage and inflammation. Thus, tumors can appear as lesions that do not heal, which enjoy the frequent presence of inflammatory cells and cytokines to heal tissue damage. In the case of chronic necrobiosis during a tumor, however, the wound does not heal, inflammation does not resolve, and instead, the tumor growth is enhanced.

Stimulation of apoptotic necrobiosis in tissues can also be pro-inflammatory and oncogenic. Chronic apoptotic necrobiosis within the liver can trigger inflammation, greater tissue damage, and an increased risk of HCC. Hepatocyte necrobiosis activates resident macrophages

(Kupe cells) to supply heptameric that stimulate resident proliferation. It is often a traditional response to repair tissue damage. Still, when the underlying cause is persistent (hepatitis viral infection, alcohol consumption, toxins, perhaps defective hoarseness), this chronic inflammation promotes tumorigenesis. Thus, acute necrobiosis may also be necessary for the elimination of tumors. In contrast, chronic necrobiosis may promote tissue damage, inflammation, and tumorigenesis. Interestingly, autophagy defects in mice cause hepatocyte toxicity, liver damage, and HCC.

Autophagy-defective embryonic tissues are impaired to remove cell corpses, which both enhance the ability to lengthen pro-inflammatory stimuli through enhanced necrobiosis and, therefore, failure to eradicate dead cells. Immortal mouse mammary epithelial cells with frequent loss of Beclin1 are cell-grown when grown as three-dimensional atmospheres, but do not contribute to inflammation and increased tumorigenesis. Apoptosis-defective tumors with autophagy defects exhibit chronic necrosis and inflammation with chronic macrophage infiltration compared to tumors with NF-dB activation and cytokine production where autophagy is intact. These findings are following autophagy promoting tumor cell survival and limiting inflammation as a non-cell autonomous means to suppress tumorigenesis. These heterogeneous tumor cell survivals promote and tumor-suppressing activities contribute to autophagy, acting as a double-edged sword within the cancer setting.

Autophagy Limits Genome Damage

Cells in mice tissues with autophagy defect accumulate damaged mitochondria and p62- and ubiquitin-containing protein aggregates, suggesting a general role for autophagy in the maintenance of cellular health through damage mitigation. Immortal somatic cell lines from autophagy-defective mice show genome damage, indicating that failure of mitigation of injury by autophagy in checkpoint-deficient cells may ultimately result in DNA mutation and chromosomal instability. Since an elevated mutation rate and genome instability promotes cancer, it increases the possibility that mitigation by autophagy and protection of the genome may be a possible tumor suppression mechanism. How autophagy protects the genome from damage is not yet clear but may result from the clearance of damaged proteins and organelles and, therefore, suppression of oxidative stress. The accumulation of either protein aggregates or damaged mitochondria is related to the increased production of reactive oxygen species (ROS). Damaged protein accumulation causes oxidative stress is not apparent but may result from increased protein depletion and isomerization during re-folding, which is an oxidation reaction. The degradation of deformed or unfolded proteins via autophagy can eliminate the need for excessive folding activity and oxidative stress.

Damaged mitochondria are a well-known source of ROS resulting from the dissolution of electron transport. ROS, in turn, mediates further organelles, protein damage, and DNA damage. Failure of protein and organelle internal control in autophagy-deficient cells can lead to a downward spiral where the persistence of damaged proteins and organelles causes ROS that damage proteins and organelles and, ultimately, the genome. If this happens frequently, the acceleration of oxidative stress may ultimately be the pathway explanation for cell damage that renders autophagy-deficient cells more tumor prone and shows the protective function of autophagy. If so, it can have a unique mechanism of suppression of tumors. It will transplant antioxidants as a protective measure where autophagy defects are predicted to predispose to cancer. Ultimately, identifying the source of ROS and whether exiled proteins or damaged organs contribute to ROS production is going to be informative.

The role of autophagic necrobiosis is in autophagy contrast to survival-promoting function supported by substantial evidence that autophagic induction necrobiosis has also been proposed as a potential tumor suppression mechanism. It follows from the observation that necrobiosis may be concurrent with the features of autophagy, which through over-expression of betanin 1, excessive stimulation of autophagy suppresses tumorigenesis. Prolonged stress and progressive autoimmunity may also eventually lead to necrobiosis. Excessive cellular damage can lead to over-stimulating autophagy and cellular self-consumption to necrobiosis. In VHDL-negative renal cell carcinoma, small molecules that promote autophagic necrobiosis are identified during a screen for synthetic lethargy with loss of VHDL. Can the approach of induction of autophagic tumor necrobiosis be added to the clinic? In vivo evidence in mammals to support these concepts is thus far limited. One obstacle to validate the concept of autophagic necrobiosis is that disrupting autophagy improves cellular survival in the sole marker. The identification, and definition, of biochemical markers for autophagic necrobiosis is going to be valuable to determine how it may differ from other types of apoptosis, necrosis, entasis, necroptosis, or necrobiosis. Also, several studies reporting the induction of autophagic necrobiosis have been performed with nonspecific pharmacological inhibitors of autophagy or apoptosis, or with RNAi-mediated knockdown of autophagy regulators. These approaches are problematic thanks to closed target effects.

In contrast, autophagic necrobiosis in Drosophila is an important tissue remodeling and resource recombination process of larval morphogenesis. A potentially similar role for hoarseness in mammalian cells during tissue remodeling is going to be important for research. One example where the stress of cellular resource recombination in mammals is senescence. The stress of oncogene activation triggers oncogene-induced senescence (OIS). This tumor suppression mechanism prevents budding tumor cells from exiting the cell cycle, cellular remodeling, and secretion of inflammatory mediators. Induces during autophagy and promotes senescence, including secretory phenotypes. The power of autophagy to turnover intracellular turnover may facilitate senescence by intracellular recycling and remodeling during the acquisition of the sense phenotype.

It would be of interest to investigate the role that autophagy-competent senescence plays in tumor suppression.

Cancer may be retinopathy. Autopage mutants play a function within the degradation of proteins. They may protect from degenerative conditions such as Parkinson's and Huntington's chorea, by inhibiting their accumulation. Accumulation of mutant huntingtin proteins and neurodegeneration is accelerated by defective autophagy and is suppressed by autophagy stimulation. Autophagy defects further accelerate the buildup of polyubiquitinated protein aggregates and neurodegeneration within the course of normal aging. Mutant protein accumulation or disease progression of retinopathy may, in general, enjoy autophagy as a mechanism to facilitate their degradation and border accumulation. Cancer is additionally a disease of mutant or overlapping protein accumulation and can be considered a type of retinopathy, where auberge mutated oncoproteins (receptor tyrosine kinases, for example) or tumor suppression proteins (p53, for example) are many The major features of the tumor are. Does autophagy suppress the formation of those proteins to limit oncogenesis?

Reduction in autophagy and protein attenuation causes abnormal accumulation of the endoplasmic reticulum (ER) chaperones and p62 that act to direct polyceratid proteins to the autophagosome for degeneration. Proteins may place a greater burden on the internal control system through higher rates of protein synthesis due to cancer protein overgrowth, mutant protein expression, or constitutive growth. Some cancers, such as myeloma, are sensitive to proteasome inhibitors, which may result in higher rates of immunoglobulin production and increased generation of unfolded proteins. Proteasome- and autophagy-mediated protein degradation may play an overlapping and complementary role in maintaining intrinsic protein control, and cancer may increase the demand for these activities to limit damage, preserving viability.

Autophagy and the double-edged sword of cancer: damage mitigation versus survival promotion

The emerging role of autophagy in cancer lies between a double-edged sword. On the one hand, autophagy enables tumor cells to tolerate stress, including hypoxic microenvironments, starvation, and doubtless therapy. Even with prolonged stress, autophagy may allow longer survival, producing dormant tumor cells that can resume growth when conditions are more favorable. This process of stress survival, lethargy, and regeneration borne by autophagy can be a serious obstacle to achieving successful cancer treatment. On the other hand, autophagy plays an important role in damage mitigation in response to anxiety that will limit tumorigenesis. By eliminating damaged proteins and organelles, and perhaps maintaining energy homeostasis through intracellular recycling, autophagy may ultimately prevent genomic damage that drives tumorigenesis. Damage mitigation can also suppress tumorigenesis by limiting chronic necrobiosis and inflammation that will promote tumorigenesis. It is easy to see how the dysregulation of autophagy that impairs cellular fitness promotes tumorigenesis. Tumor cells can adapt and grow in response to selective pressures and become progressively more malleable to their human hosts, which makes it difficult to treat cancer. Autophagy may suppress this development while maintaining homeostatic conditions. Although the survival of tumor cells can also be increased by autophagy, it can be repaired by damage mitigation action. In tumor cells with inactive autophagy, increased gene damage, and decreased survival due to market tumor growth and chronic inflammation may also be inconsistent. Subsequent challenges are to use this theory guiding principles to examine autophagy modulation within the setting of cancer therapy, keeping in mind that tumors with autophagy intact may respond differently from those with autophagy. Is. Another challenge is to accept functional autophagy status in tumors to direct acceptable therapy.

As autophagy inhibits the survival of metabolic stress with autophagy, a survival pathway used by tumor cells may have to tolerate metabolic stress, autophagy inhibitors are expected to be useful for the treatment of cancer. Autophagy inhibitors are particularly attractive because they will target tumor cells in hypoxic tumor areas that are resistant to therapy, especially radiation. Additionally, tumor cells within the process of metastasizing may also be specifically implicated in autophagy, supporting approaches to abrogate autophagy in early progression and, therefore, the adjuvant setting. Although some deaths can result from autophagy inhibitors causing loss of survival in stress, they can also hinder dormancy and recovery.

It is unlikely that autophagy inhibitors are going to be useful for cancer therapy as a single agent because only a subset of tumor cells undergo autophagy. Because many cancer practitioners induce autophagy, they induce damage (cytotoxic chemotherapy), metabolic stress (angiogenesis inhibitors, 2-deoxyglucose), or growth signaling pathways (targeted non-cytotoxic, kinase inhibitors). Factors promote deprivation or starvation. Inhibitors would be expected to reinforce the cytotoxicity of those agents. mTOR inhibitors induce autophagy, and if it protects from stress, their full therapeutic benefit will be realized in association with autophagy inhibitors. The approach here is to damage stress adaptation and to increase damage by inhibiting autophagy. It would be important to induce acute rather than chronic necrobiosis and inflammation that would be countercyclical. The downside to the current approach is that damage mitigation and loss of potential tumor suppression activity. This may not be a problem if the induction of stress with inhibition of autophagy growth sufficiently kills all tumor cells. Normal tissue must address potentially fatal accidents, although the metabolic stress inherent in the tumor may provide a therapeutic window.

The inhibition of apoptosis, dormancy, and regeneration would be an alternative approach specifically targeting survival, latency, and regeneration mechanisms, which work together or together with autophagy. For example, disabling apoptosis should reduce the inactivation and acquisition of uptake. Although autophagy inhibition stimulates apoptosis, a selected apoptotic mechanism, may be responsible for the survival and regeneration of latent cells that will be identified. An anti-apoptotic Bcl-2 inhibitor is in clinical trials to market tumor cell apoptosis. Metabolic stress triggers apoptosis that is disrupted by Bcl-2, requires a pro-apoptotic Bam, and is indicated through the core pro-apoptotic regulators Box and Back. Whether BCL-2 is additionally required for the viability of latent and regenerated tumor cells should be assessed. Defining the mechanisms that control latency and regeneration may reveal novel targets downstream of autism, and it is probably valuable to inhibit these processes. Inactivation- and regeneration-specific inhibitors may have the advantage of maintaining the protective, damage mitigation function of autophagy.

Development and evaluation of autophagy inhibitors in cancer therapy cancer therapy

It should be possible to develop autophagy inhibitors specific to because of kinases (Atg1 / Unc-51-like-kinase 1/2/3, Vps34), proteases, and two ubiquitous-like conjugation systems. Are they regulating the activation of autophagy and autophagosome formation? There are also signaling pathways, both motor-dependent and dependent, that control the activation of autophagy that would be targeted. For example, elongation factor-2 kinase (EEF-2 kinase), which is downstream from mTOR, promotes autophagy-mediated survival of glioblastoma and is therefore expected to be a clinically useful GEF-2 kinase inhibitor. Are going to be

Autophagosomes have poorly understood mechanisms to target proteins and organelles that are likely to have additional targets. Signaling pathways that promote autophagy are also good candidates for inhibitory development. Currently, hydroxychloroquine (HCQ), which blocks lysosome acidification and autophagosome degradation, is out as an autophagy inhibitor that would be able to assess the utility of this approach. A variety of clinical trials have been initiated and are currently recruiting patients with solid and hematopoietic tumors to investigate this. Most of those trials are combinations of HCQ with cytotoxic chemotherapy, targeted therapies for metabolic stress, or with the general hypothesis that autophagy may be a mechanism of therapeutic resistance and that HCQ will increase cytotoxicity by abrogation of auxopathy. As shown in Table 2, most of those studies combine HCQ with a more standard cancer therapy expected to induce autophagy. If there is a therapeutic benefit to preventing autophagy for cancer therapy, these tests should reveal. Although HCQ is not an exclusive autophagy inhibitor, it is relatively non-cytotoxic. It blocks the flow through the autophagy pathway by inhibiting the terminal lysosome degradation step. It remains to be demonstrated whether HCQ can block lysis in human tumors in vivo and if either the genetic makeup of the tumor affects this response or not. To the present end, identification of biomarkers and signatures, reflecting the functional autophagy status that detects therapeutic modulation of autophagy in human tumors, will require development.

Efficacy of HCQ and chloroquine (CQ) in models preclinical the efficacy of autophagy inhibition with CQ and CQ has begun to be evaluated in animal models. Human cancer cells and characteristics, and, therefore results are encouraging. My-driven lymphoma enhances the potency of either p53 or alkylating agents for tumor necrobiosis during HCQ and a mouse model for autophagy inhibition. CQ, Atm-telangiectasia and n My-transgenic mice that model human Burkitt lymphoma impose spontaneous lymphomas in model Ataxia telangiectasia and n My-transgenic mice. However, CQ did not prevent spontaneous lymphomas in p53 deficient mice. The mechanism of CQ-mediated tumor cell toxicity was following the promotion of lysosomal stress and p53-dependent and apoptosis-independent tumor necrobiosis. Thus, CQ may increase the activity, promoting the death of a standard tumor suppression pathway to prevent cancer development. CQ also promotes neoplastic cell death in association with chronic myelogenous leukemia (CML) cell lines and the HDC inhibitor hydroxamic acid (SAHA) and the first CML to express wild-type and imatinib-resistant mutant types of Bar-Abl. Cells. The synergy of CQ and SAHA was related to induction. It was enhanced by the lysosomal protease cathepsin D, suggesting that CQ and autophagy inhibition promote tumor necrobiosis by a lysosome-driven process. As the CQ and HCQ blocks flow through the autophagy pathway in the lysosomal degradation phase, it would be of interest to coincide and contrast with the effectiveness of blocked autophagy initiation. Collectively, these findings suggest that autophagy inhibition may enhance the anticancer activity of chemotherapy and endogenous tumor suppression mechanisms, which regulate tumor regression and limit spontaneous tumor growth.

The pathway of protein degradation for cancer chemotherapy There Changing Are two main protein degradation systems in cells, autophagy, which may be a mechanism for the degradation of bulk proteins in lysosomes, and hence the proteasome pathway, tagged with polyubiquitin There may be a mechanism for degradation of individual proteins. In the cells.

These two pathways may be partially complementary or interdependent for protein degradation, and inhibition of the protease pathway induces autophagy and inhibition of autophagy leads to the formation of polyubiquitin proteins. Furthermore, autophagy avoids toxicity, while autophagy defects confer sensitivity to proteasome inhibition, which supports the compensatory nature of those protein degradation pathways. There is also evidence that polyubiquitin-containing protein aggregates can prevent proteasome-mediated degradation by inhibiting promotes above. Predictions are that inhibiting both the proteasome and the autophagy degradation pathway may be more toxic to cancer cells, particularly those with high rates of protein synthesis that secrete those immunoglobulins (multiple myeloma). Indeed, myeloma is sensitive to the proteasome inhibitor Velde, which is approved by the FDA to treat this cancer. The validity of mixing HCQ to reinforce Velde in myeloma is being evaluated within the clinic. Similarly, the histone deacetylase HDAC6, which binds polyubiquitinated proteins and promotes the degradation of autophagy-mediated proteins, and the inhibition of HDAC activity with SAHA synergize with Velde to kill myeloma. Thus, inhibiting both the proteasome and autophagy pathways may also be an important approach for the treatment of cancer.

Since the stimulation of autophagy for cancer chemotherapeutics predisposes to autophagy defects to cancer and other diseases, the possibility of stimulating autophagy as a disease prevention measure is promising. In a model of neurodegeneration, inhibiting autophagy accelerates disease progression, while stimulating autophagy with MTOR inhibitors or other autophagy stimulants or by increasing HDAC6 expression delays disease progression. Investigations are on whether this strategy is going to be effective for cancer prevention. Non-specific means such as caloric restriction and the exciting autophagy of fasting can improve human health and suppress cancer. At the same time, consumption of additional nutrition that is harmful to suppress autophagy is considered. It would be of interest to investigate whether these activities are often attributed to the modulation of autophagy.

Autophagy defects in mice cause diseases such as steatohepatitis and HCC. Patients with steatohepatitis are at risk of developing HCC and are a candidate group to investigate autophagy stimulation for cancer prevention. CQ can suppress spontaneous, oncogene activation-driven lymphomas in mice, suggesting that inhibition of autophagy may also be a prevention strategy. Extending the suppressive activity of the tumor, like p53, with autophagy inhibitors may also be more beneficial during this setting. In contrast, steatohepatitis is a clinical protein internal control failure and may rather enjoy autophagy stimulation. With steatohepatitis, tissue damage and therefore, the resulting inflammation promotes HCC that will be suppressed by autophagy stimulation. Stimulation of autophagy abolishes p62-containing Mallory bodies induced by proteome inhibition, p62 accumulation is responsible for liver toxicity and teases in autophagy-deficient mice. Low baicalin levels and low autophagy also worsen disease in HCC. Maybe that's the reason. Combination cancer therapy targets many. Distinct pathways are important for treatment and therefore, the autophagy pathway provides novel ways to reinforce therapy.

Chapter 5: Useful Tips and The Right Mindset to Start Intermittent Fasting

If you are fasting (or thinking about starting fasting), you must adopt the right mentality.

I've put together some suggestions and strategies that will help you on this path.

Easy Tricks to Deceive Hunger

Hot-Drink Method

I know when I'm eating fewer calories, I crave everything. Some people get angry while fasting. Who cares, this trick is dirty, and it works.

If you are feeling like you are going crazy and are getting something to eat, this is not the time (usually with a full day of fasting), then you must resort to something else Would like

Enter: a delicious, hot drink.

My personal favorite is JM ax cocoa (which I will be able to give below the recipe since such a gentleman), but coffee or tea also works.

Sometimes, if the cravings are crazy, I'll have 2 or 3 of those hot bags.

- JM ax Hot Chocolates
- Boiling Water
- 1 Teaspoon Chocolate
- 9 Liquid Stevia
- Drops BCCAs Method

If you have ever fasted all day, you recognize that you will simply get the hunger spikes almost exactly on time that you normally eat. Your body knows when it wants to eat and can find you. It is often caused by a tactile hormone called Ghrelin. The big news is that if you don't eat after this Ghrelin spike, your body will spike another hormone: Somatotropin.

Everyone knows how dangerous somatotropin is to fat loss, so I'll leave it at that.

If this hunger spike causes your wish that you are dying or going crazy, then the BCAAs are for you.

BCAAS is a calorie-free nutrient that will baffle your body, thinking that you have eaten just a touch, and therefore will reduce appetite. Sometimes taking BCAAs that you eat normally will help increase appetite.

Before we all get lovey dove, and someone tells me that they stood at my door with their hands on my waist and kissed me as they meant it; Let's just keep it PG.

While spreading your hunger, you will just sit there as if you are a 3rd party and analyze it. Ask yourself questions like, "Am I really hungry, or is this just a sign that baffles my mind?" Sit there and realize what you don't want to eat. Do not believe food; just believe in your body and make it work. Soon, you will see that the appetite suddenly decreases.

Keep-Busy

Often the thought and desire to eat can make your waiting difficult.

Take advantage of it and stay busy. Work, do a puzzle, call a boyfriend, or read a book.

Sleep-It-Off

My friend Tim inspired me to make it. Whenever I feel about this story, it makes me laugh.

Last year, I had a bunch of classes with Tim so that we would sit together. One day, he did not show up until our last class (6 hours after the primary one). He sits down, and here we have our conversation:

"Tim, you're too late, man."

"Yes, I tried to talk of fasting you are talking about on your blog ..."

"It has nothing to do with why you are 6 hours late." Dumb excuse, man.
"

No, don't hold on to you. I didn't eat, so I all felt tired and tired and slept like that for 5 hours. I think my body needs food alternatively, here Till I have no energy. "

Yes, this conversation happened. It is good to understand that hungry children in Africa never suffer because they are sleeping all the time.

All joking aside, this Ba the conversation got me thinking. If you only sleep on the day you're fasting, nap within the afternoon, then it loves it's never been.

It's like sleeping and juggling on an extended car-ride Se is like waking up to my destination... and everyone likes magic.

These were many objections to a nutritionist who, during a consultation four years ago, concluded a 3-month intermittent fasting protocol. Leads to Nutritionists were adamant that intermittent fasting would cause me the most trouble, which weight gain as well as weight loss, an unhealthy diet, constant fatigue. And poor concentration, calls a couple.

Although I had my doubts, thirty minutes after taking a nutritionist's note about the benefits of international fasting, I decided to self-experiment and made it available.

The next day I skipped breakfast, broke my fast at noon, and ate my last meal at 7 pm. For the next three months, I can follow the current protocol type of a trooper.

On the last day of the scheduled three-month period, I walked into a field gym, took off my shoes and put both of my feet on a white weight scale.

I did not expect results (in fact, I did not track my weight change during the three months). Then, I saw the shape numbers go up and up, then it stopped. And I was shocked.

I had lost 22 pounds (10 kg).

I got accustomed and immediately started to end three months of intermittent fasting. In those three months at least a year, then two years and today, after four years of intermittent fasting, I would say that this is one of the simplest decisions of my life.

Here are eleven good and bad lessons that I have learned from intermittent fasting, along with some insights that will be useful to you.

Good and bad lessons from 4 years of intermittent fasting 1. Intermittent fasting is not a 'starvation' diet; it is a healthy lifestyle.

Most people I have intermittently shared the philosophy of fasting, usually commenting by saying, "Oh, yes, I did that, before you mean to starve yourself to reduce the right is?"

It cannot be beyond reality.

Intermittent fasting is not a diet. It is a pattern of eating. Or to be more specific, it is a lifestyle that will last a lifetime.

And as a lifestyle, it is important to track and measure your progress.

I have personally used flexible measuring tapes to urge accurate measurements of my body, which the scales often miss. Lightweight digital scales are also useful for tracking weight loss, just confirm yourself to live in an equal time of day to avoid wrong results.

Listen to your body for what to eat.

One of the usual inquiries about intermittent fasting is what rotates to eat during the protocol.

From my experience, any balanced healthy diet will suffice. However, a diet like the 'Blue Zone' diet can help maintain weight loss, improve mental performance and health.

The most important lesson I have learned about what I eat is to focus on my body and eat to suit my needs.

For example, if you feel tired and dry after eating rice or cereal, you will try to eat more vegetables instead. If you are feeling more energetic after doing this, your body's way is to stick to vegetables and avoid the intake of high carbohydrate foods.

Therefore, I am a strong advocate against a 'fixed' diet.

As we get older, our body constantly changes, as well, eating equal meals a day increases the chances of developing food intolerance and diseases.

Thankfully, I found this concept of 'eating with your body in mind' while reading the work of internationally renowned Holistic Health Specialist, Paul Czech — specifically, in his book Eat to Move and Be Healthy.

The important lesson here is to constantly listen to your body and experiment with different foods for optimal health.

Proven Truths That Will Help You Maintain Your Goal

Intermittent fasting simplifies your life

Before practicing intermittent fasting, I would spend hours cooking, cooking and cooking six meals each day. This tedious routine caused inconsistencies with my weight training routine and its consequences had to suffer for me.

Nowadays, my life can be a lot simpler.

I eat one or two staple meals a day - about to live without eating - and still make steady progress towards achieving my health goals.

Intermittent fasting protocol simplifies life by reducing the amount of selection you make.

Expect your results after one year.

During my first year of intermittent fasting, I lost weight, shed an honest chunk of fat and leaned into the simplest shape of my life. But after my first year, my weight and fat loss decreased significantly, and so the results were reduced over the years.

It is sensible since if your body is harmful to your health, a lot of such facts can be lost.

Be sure to keep track of your intermittent fasting progress on a spreadsheet or a robust notebook for future reference.

Intermittent fasting plus high-intensity interval training equals rapid fat loss.

If you want to reduce fat as soon as possible, I recommend you do any type of training with high intensity.

For example, once I started intermittent fasting, I offered 10 minutes of sprinting three times per week, as well as weekly football matches.

You can do any type of exercise, i.e., swimming, skipping, jogging, increase the intensity until you get out after every workout.

Also, high-intensity interval training on an empty stomach further accelerates fat loss (in my experience). I am not exactly sure about the science of why training in fasting conditions can help with fat loss, so I would recommend you experiment with it.

Intuitively, it is sensible why it might work as an intermittent fast, helping to limit calorie intake, while high-intensity interval training burns calories. Over time, your total daily calorie intake drops significantly, and more fat is shed from your body.

Intermittent fasting can improve your discipline, focus, and productivity.

During my fasting window, by 1 pm on most days, if I wake up once, I buy more work than breakfast. Once I break my fast with the primary food, my energy levels decrease, then I lose focus and feel lethargic.

For this reason, I have set my most important task before I break my fast. This enables me to match my peak energy levels with my top priorities, leading to higher levels of productivity.

Another observation that I have noticed is that one-day fasting habit has greatly improved my discipline during the rest of my life. Once I made a habit of intermittent fasting, I developed the will to start new habits - eating healthy, sleeping fast, reading more than one. This is often a feature of keystone habits.

Intermittent fasting can reduce your discipline, focus, and productivity.

This may seem contrary to this point, but if you think about it, hunger can cause irritability. In other words, when it becomes easier to fast, then lose focus and get excited thanks to a severe stomach.

Therefore, it is so important to focus on your body, rather than sticking to a hard and fast diet.

I have noticed that every day is a sweet spot to stop your fasting window - a period. If you break, you're fast too quickly, you will miss the energy that may be used to do more work. If you break, you're fast too late, you will start getting excited and concentrate during the day.

Every day is different, so confirm the experiment and find out what works for you.

Intermittent fasting can make your diet worse

Following my point, when you are extremely hungry and break your fast, it is easy to eat unhealthy or nutritious empty food.

This has been one of my biggest challenges with intermittent fasting. It takes human discipline to fast for a day. But it takes supernatural discipline to fast and maintain a clean diet a day.

The reason is that when you are fasting, your body is low on sugar and energy. It also craves high carbohydrate foods with sugar.

If you have achieved your weight loss goals without eating a clean diet, at the end of the day, it can be harmful to your health.

The best way I have stopped this overarching trend after breaking the fast is to style my environment for fulfillment and drink more and more water throughout the day.

Intermittent fasting can contribute to muscle loss and gain.

During my second year of intermittent fasting, I injured my lower back while squatting and had to stay away from the weight indefinitely.

Therefore, I replaced my weight training with Pilates and stretching exercises. Additionally, I started a body detox program, which included removing high-carbohydrate foods from my diet for a few months.

Within a few weeks, my muscles were significantly reduced, which my clothes no longer fit. The detox program and intermittent fasting protocols significantly reduced my daily calorie intake, causing muscle damage.

Once I recovered from the injury and resumed the weight training program - increasing my carbohydrate intake - within a few months, I regained my physique and regained muscle.

The main lesson here is that calorie intake matters a lot!

Intermittent fasting can be a tool to scale back calorie intake.

Like any newbie, during the primary year of intermittent fasting, I believed that I had discovered the magic formula to lose weight and lean. I can teach everyone how intermittent fasting was the only thanks to achieving their health goals because it worked so well on my behalf.

Over the years, as I have experimented with intermittent fasting, I have found that the most frequent reason why intermittent fasting works so well for weight loss is that it helps regain the amount of time - And thus - the amount of food you will eat.

The less food you eat, the fewer calories you eat, and therefore you lose weight.

This is simple mathematics. There is nothing magical about it.

Those who intermittently try fasting and failure lament that it does not work. But, in most cases, it is because they do not track calories properly.

Intermittent fasting is just another tool to assist you in increasing your calorie intake. If you choose to eat food after an extended fast, you still gain yourself more weight than you lost. Will do!

Intermittent fasting is not an excuse to enjoy your favorite frozen dessert or chocolate cookie regardless of the world.

By the time you make sure that the total calories consumed are a small amount you maneuver and live with every day, you will reduce and burn fat.

Intermittent fasting should not stop you from enjoying your life.

The biggest lesson I have learned during my 4-year journey of intermittent fasting is to avoid worrying about being perfect and luxated in life, with no progress towards my weight and fitness goals.

During the primary year of intermittent fasting, I refused to interrupt my fast outside my eating window.

I would travel to new places over the holidays, remembering the experiences of eating new food from different cultures as I used to do "intermittently."

I often saw people who did not live as healthy lifestyles as I did and held to a rigid intermittent fasting protocol.

But over time, I have learned that there is more to life than losing weight, gaining muscle, and getting in shape. Certainly, I still work towards achieving my health goals every day, but I can't beat myself if I ruin myself.

Chapter 6: The Most Common Mistakes to Avoid

You Are Jumping Too Fast into Intermittent Fasting

The biggest reason most diets fail is that they are so extreme a departure from our normal, natural way of eating that they often find it impossible to take care of. Just an idea, but if you are a new IF and are familiar with eating every two hours, maybe don't throw yourself into a difficult 24-hour fast from hell. If you are adamant about the concept of fasting, start with the initial 12/12 method where you are fasting for 12 hours per day and eating within a 12-hour window. It is probably on the verge of what you want to do anyway, and who knows, it will be the only (if that too) to follow up with sustainable thanks.

You Are Choosing The Wrong Plan for Your Lifestyle

Then, do not set yourself up for misery that assimilates your style by signing up for something you have identified. If you are an evening owl, do not decide to start your fast at 6 pm. If you are a daily gym-goer who Instagram's your WOD every morning and is not ready to sacrifice your daily spin, do not select one. Consider taking calories seriously for a few days each week. Is banned from. You must do one if you want any habit of staying.

You Are Eating an Excessive Amount During The Eating Window

This is one that the most common trap I can expect is that people come with IF. If you have chosen a very restrictive rule, which leaves you to hang the Air Force for hours of the day, the clock immediately says, "It's time to eat," you're likely to travel in the weeds. Research shows that restrictive diets often do not work because we are emotionally (and physically) stressed that once we allow ourselves to eat, we go wild during the absence of deprivation and Hunt more. Any diet you have taken together with your next meal can be a recipe for a binge, so confirm that you are not allowing yourself to feel unnecessarily hungry for a long period.

You Are Not Eating Enough During The Dinner Window

Yes, not eating enough is an additional legal explanation for weight gain, and I'll tell you why. In addition to setting yourself up for a rebound, as we discussed with the previous common IF mistake, not eating enough will soften your muscles, slowing your metabolism. Without that metabolic muscle mass, you will be sabotaging your ability to lose fat (never mind losing) in the future. The challenge with IF is that because you are eating conforming to some arbitrary cosmic rules rather than paying attention to your body's innate signals, it is difficult to understand your real needs. If you are adamant about dieting, make sure to talk to a registered dietitian to help you assess your nutritional needs.

What Are You Ignoring in Favor Of?

IF can be a time-intensive diet, and most "plans" provide no clear rules about the type of food you eat during your "eating window." But this is not an excuse to subsist on a diet of French-fried potatoes, milkshakes, and beer. Fasting is not magic. In addition to some small metabolic benefits, its primary effect on weight loss (if it has one at all) is essentially supported by the fact that you are limiting you're eating hours and thus reducing your chances of calorie consumption. Have been.

If you choose the wrong type of foods, unfortunately, this effect often reduces quickly. Shift your approach to the idea of treating yourself during your "limited" feasts to indulge in nutrient-dense, nutritious foods during those times. We recommend that every meal or snack has a combination of saturated fiber, protein, and good fats to help carry you through your fasting phase.

You Are Not Drinking Enough

Your intermittent fasting diet may require you to avoid food. Still, water must pass, especially since you are missing hydration when you regularly get it from foods such as fruits and vegetables.

Dehydration can cause muscle cramps, headaches, and reduced appetite, so always confirm that you are sucking H_2O between (and during) feasts.

All the principles followed and still struggling? That's not you; This is a possibility of anorexia. Research suggests that there is a 31 percent drop in the rate of intermittent fasting. In contrast, research on a diet has generally suggested that the maximum amount fails as a 95 percent diet. Your body tries to focus more on what the person tells you, rather than what the watch says, and you must be more insistent on meeting your body's needs.

Chapter 7: Helpful Recommendations, Risks and Example of a Balanced Meal Plan

Generally, intermittent fasting is safe for many people, but you also understand the risks.

It is also an honest time to mention that your doctor should not consult this lesson and that you should always consult your doctor before planning any fast and especially extended fasting (more than 24 hours).

Now that we have made it clear, here are several cases (but it will not be limited) that do not go well with intermittent fasting:

If you have diabetes, if you are taking medications for vital signs, remember the condition.,

If you have a disease, do not sleep if you do not sleep, if you are under 18, you should be more careful if you are practicing extended fasting., Which is being counted on the source you follow, being fasted continuously for any of the 24, 48 or 72 hours. The consensus is that any fast over 72 hours should be performed under strict medical supervision.

Intermittent Fasting 18/6:

Do for 18 hours and eat 6 hours. Like almost the above, if you choose the 18/6 intermittent fasting schedule, you should fast for 18 hours and eat your food for 6 hours. Should be confined to the window.

This is just two hours of fasting every day, except for an initial fast, these 2 hours can make all the difference.

Therefore, we recommend starting at a minimum of 16/8 months until you go to 18/6, as you will have a way more pleasant, and this is an important element between leaving and not doing.

Intermittent Fasting 5:2 Aka Fat Diet

How it works: 2 days restricts calories to 500-600 per week, 5 days per week.

Intermittent fasting 5:2, normally allows you to eat 5 days per week and restricts your calorie intake to 500. 600 per day during the opposite 2 days. When choosing your fasting days, limit the mind that there should be at least one regular eating day in between.

Please note that your results depend on what you eat during the 5 days of non-fasting, thus staying nutritious and with a complete diet for maximum results.

Intermittent Fasting 20/4 Aka Warrior Diet:

How it works: Eat for 20 hours and eat for 4h.

Unlike other methods, following the 20/4 intermittent fasting schedule, you can eat some raw fruits and vegetables and some lean. Proteins during the 20-hour fast period.

This fasting schedule is based on the thinking that our ancestors would spend their days hunting and gathering and then feasting in the dark. Therefore the 4-hour eating window will be within the evening, and you should follow a sequence of eating specific food groups: starting with vegetables, protein, and fat and eating carbs while you are still hungry.

OMAD Fasting Aka 23/1:

How to have: Eat 23h. Take a fast and another popular fasting program is named One Day Meal (OMAD).

This is what it appears like - you select a time during a day that is best suited for you and you only have a meal of the day.

I know what you're thinking - isn't he almost hungry? And yes, you're right - an OMAD diet should not be avoided on the way to achieving a minimum of 1200 calories during one meal.

Thus, if you choose this 23/1 fast - confirm that your food can be hearty and nutritious.

HR Fast Aka Eat Stop Eat:

Fast for twenty-four hours. During a 24-hour fast (popularized by the Eat Stop Eat method, you should fast for twenty-four hours 1-2 days every week and normally eat on other days. In this way, you should reduce the overall calorie intake in CA calories by 10%. Should be reduced and therefore reduced.

Aqua Declaration Diet:

Do once a month for 24 hours.

As mentioned earlier, extended or prolonged fasting usually, but it means. Fasting for 24 and 96 hours.

Some Examples of a Balanced Daily Meal Plan

It is not recommended to try it more than once a month and anything above 48-72 hours of fasting should be done under doctor's supervision.

- Breakfast: Spinach Parmesan baked eggs
- Lunch: Oven-Crispy fish Tacos.
- Dinner: Turkey Burrito Skillet
- Snack: was Bitrate suggest chocolate (two sections)

- Breakfast: Hummus Breakfast Bowl
- Lunch: Baked Lemon Salmon And asparagus foil packs
- Dinner: Chicken and broccoli fried
- Snack: Coddled egg

- Breakfast: 4-ingredient protein pancakes
- Lunch: Wild cod
- Dinner: Honey garlic shrimp fried
- Snack: Almonds (suggestions 12-14)

- Breakfast: Ham and Egg breakfast cup
- Lunch: Sweet potato and turkey Skillet
- Dinner: savory Lemon White Fish Filial
- Snack: two stalks of celery

- Breakfast: No-bake oatmeal raisin Energy bits
- Lunch: Ground Turkey, olives, cucumber Feta Seth quinoa salad
- Dinner: Skinny salmon, black, and cashews Bowl
- Snack: 1 cup of fresh strawberries

Chapter 8: Recipes for Intermittent Fasting

Sweet Potato Breakfast Hash

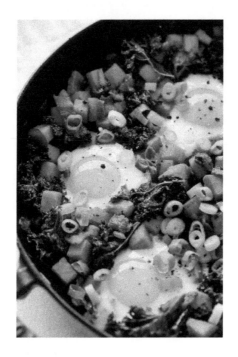

Ingredients

- 2 large sweet potatoes, peeled and minced,
- 3 tablespoons vegetable oil
- 1/2 teaspoon kosher salt
- 1/4 teaspoon ground white pepper

- 1 tbsp apple vinegar
- 2 cloves minced garlic
- 1 tablespoon honey
- 1/4 cup yellow onion, small
- 1/4 cup green bell pepper, small
- 8 ounces low-sodium sulfate-free ham, Dusted small
- 1 tablespoon juice
- 1 avocado, peel, pit removed, and small

Instructions

- Hot oven to 450 degrees. Line a baking sheet with foil.
- Mix submerged sweet potato, 1/2 tbsp vegetable oil, salt, and pepper and spread in a good layer on a baking sheet. About a quarter of an hour or until the potatoes turn tender and just begin to brown.
- Meanwhile, in a small bowl, mix apple vinegar, garlic, and honey. Whisking constantly, add 1 tbsp of vegetable oil. Until well combined
- In a large pan over medium heat, heat the remaining vegetable oil. When hot, add onion and sweet chili. Cook until the onions begin to melt and add the ham and the cooked potatoes. Cook until the ham starts to brown. Remove from heat and stir within apple vinegar sauce.
- Combine juice and avocado. Gently stir in the hash. Serve hot!
- Optional tip: Top with extra protein and a spilled egg for a full meal!

No-Bake Oatmeal Raisin Energy Bytes

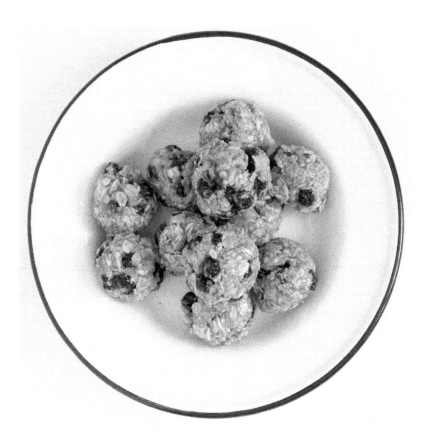

Ingredients

- 1 cup dry oats
- 1/4 cup spread
- 2 tablespoons honey
- 1/4 cup semi-sweet mini chocolate chips
- 1/4 cup raisins
- 1/4 cup peanuts,

- 1/2 teaspoon ground cinnamon
- 1 Scoop. Vanilla Protein Powder (we use Burt's Beats Protein Powder)

Instructions

- Mix all ingredients and mix properly until the mixture is well mixed and sticky.
- Roll into 1-inch balls and place on a parchment-lined baking sheet. Keep within the refrigerator for about half an hour or until firm. Store covered and refrigerated in an airtight container.

Ham and Egg Breakfast Cup

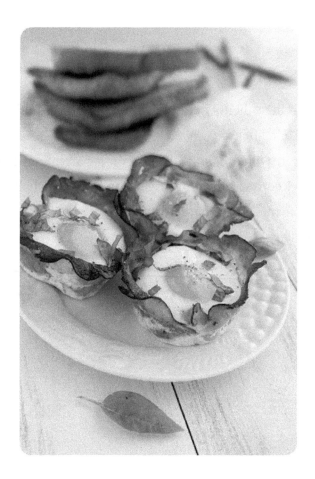

Ingredients

- 12 thin slices All-natural and low-sodium ham
- 3 eggs
- 1/2 cup skimmed milk
- 2 green onions, sliced

Instructions

- Whites Preheat oven to 350 degrees.
- Lightly spray the muffin tin with non-stick spray. Press each ham slice through the muffin pan, forming a cup shape.
- In a bowl, whisk together eggs, egg whites, and milk. Stir within the scallion and pour into the ham cup until about 3/4 full. Bake for about 20 minutes, until the eggs are fully set. Remove and allow to cool slightly before serving.! As a pleasure!

4-Ingredients Protein Pancakes

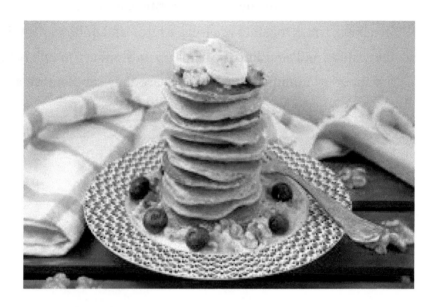

Ingredients

- 1/2 cup mashed banana
- 3 egg whites
- 1/4 teaspoon levant
- 1 scoop vanilla protein powder (we used thy protein powder, low-carb and gluten-free)

Instructions

- All ingredients during a bowl Mix until smooth,
- lightly sprayed. Skillet with non-stick spray and heat over medium heat. Pour 1/4 cup of the batter into the pan. Cook for

about 3 to 4 minutes, or until the pancakes begin to bubble within the center. Flip carefully and cook for an additional 2 to three minutes. Once cooked, remove the pancake from the pan and repeat the method until all the batter is used. In the middle of baking pancakes, spray the skillet as needed with non-stick spray.

- Top with fresh fruit, honey, or your favorite nut butter!! As a pleasure!

Hummus Breakfast Bowl

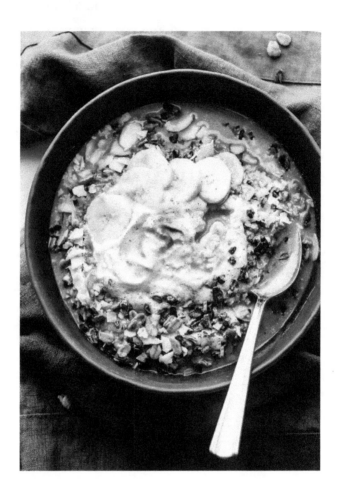

Ingredients

- 2 tablespoons bell peppers, minced meat (any color)
- 1 cup bananas, stems removed, roughly chopped leftover,
- 1/4 cup romp small
- 1 tablespoon vegetable oil
- 1/4 cup rice or quinoa (cooked)

- 1 tablespoon hummus
- 2 egg whites
- 1 teaspoon sunflower seeds

Instructions

- Heat vegetable oil in a large pan on medium heat. Add fennel as soon as it gets hot.
- Sauté the kaput for 3-4 minutes and then add tomatoes and chilies. Cook for 4-5 minutes.
- Lightly beat the egg and slowly add the bud and chili. Scramble the eggs until they run away.
- Place rice or quinoa along with vegetables and eggs at the bottom of a serving bowl. Spoon the hummus on top and sprinkle with sunflower seeds.! As a pleasure!

Spinach Parmesan Baked Egg Recipe

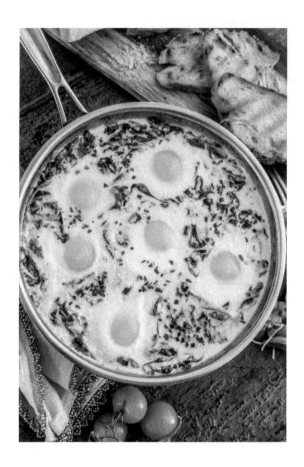

Ingredients

- 2 tablespoons vegetable oil
- 2 cloves garlic, minced
- 4 cups baby spinach
- 1/2 cup fat-free grated cheese
- 4 eggs

- 1 small tomato, small

Instructions

- Preheat the oven to 350 degrees. Spray 8 inches by 8-inch casserole dish with nonstick spray.
- In a large pan, heat the vegetable oil over medium heat. Once hot, add spinach and garlic. Stir the spinach until the spinach has wilted. Remove from heat and turn off any excess liquid. Stir within the cottage cheese and spoon the mixture into a fine layer within the casserole dish.
- Make four small partitions within the spinach for the eggs. Crack one egg into each part. Bake for 15 to 20 minutes until the egg whites are mostly set. Remove from the oven and let cool for about 5 minutes then sprinkle with tomatoes. Serve and Enjoy!

Conclusion

Thank you for making it through to the end of Intermittent Fasting for Women Over 50, let's hope it was informative and able to provide you with all of the tools you need to achieve your goals whatever they may be.

It is always good to consult a professional health care professional before making a dietary change, even if you are only changing the time when eating. They will help you determine if intermittent fasting will be beneficial for you. This is often particularly important for prolonged fasting, during which vitamin and mineral deficiency may occur. It is important to know that our bodies are incredibly intelligent. If food is limited to one meal, the body can increase appetite. Therefore, the subsequent food has a lower calorie content, and metabolism is also disrupted to match calorie consumption. Intermittent fasting has many potential health benefits, but it should not be assumed that if it is strictly followed, it is bound to prevent heavyweight loss and the occurrence or progression of the disease. This is a useful approach, but many tools may have to be implemented to help achieve and maintain optimal health.

Finally, if you found this book useful in any way, a review is always appreciated!

CPSIA information can be obtained
at www.ICGtesting.com
Printed in the USA
BVHW041202131120
593256BV00009B/123